Title: The Ji 擠 form of tai chi power compared with Bruce Lee's One-inch-punch

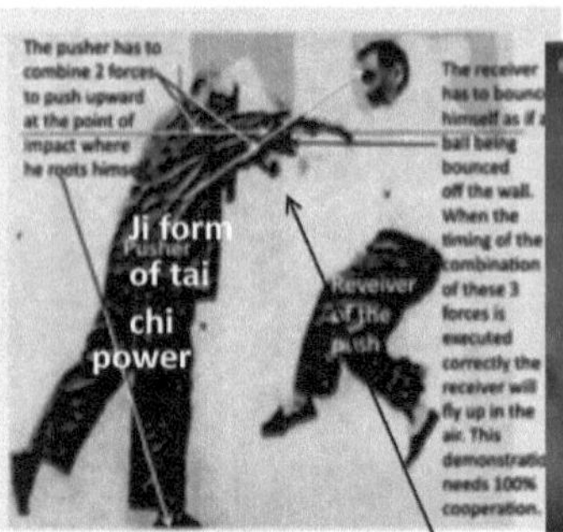

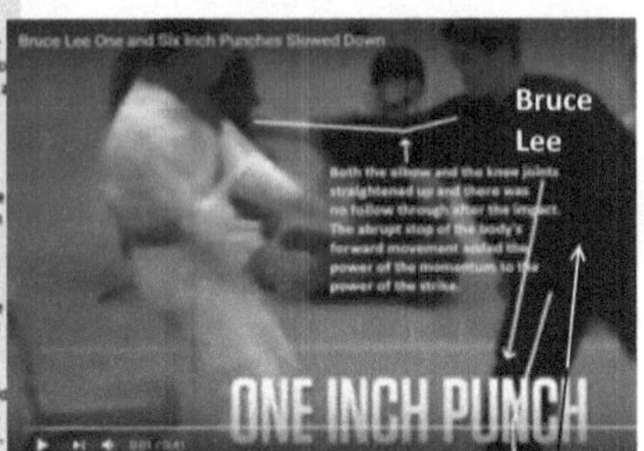

Using the 擠 Ji form of tai chi power to push someone up in the air

The same principle is used by Bruce Lee in his 1 and 6 inch punches.

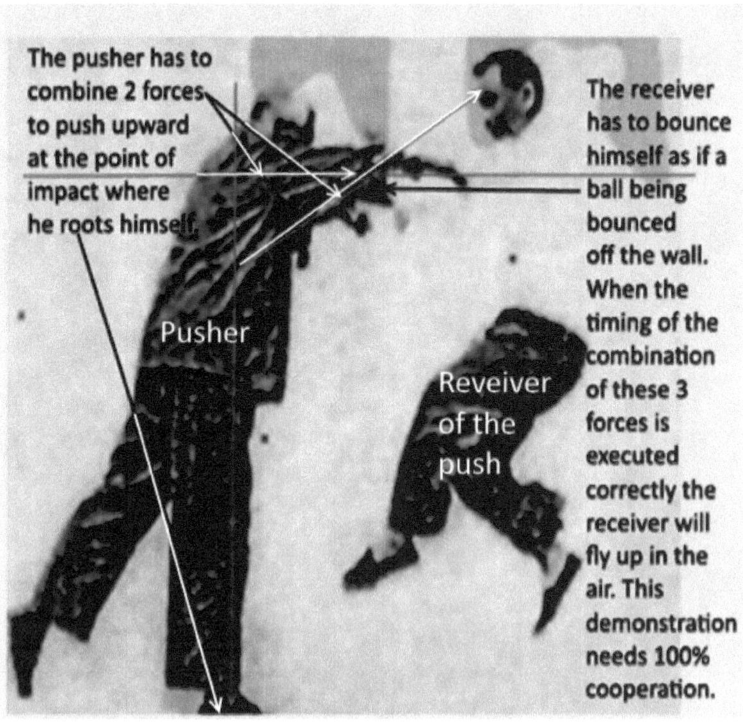
The pusher has to
combine 2 forces
to push upward
at the point of
impact where
he roots himself.
Pusher
The receiver
has to bounce
himself as if a
ball being
bounced
off the wall.
When the
timing of the
combination
of these 3
forces is
executed
correctly the
receiver will
fly up in the
air. This
demonstration
needs 100%
cooperation.
Reveiver
of the
push

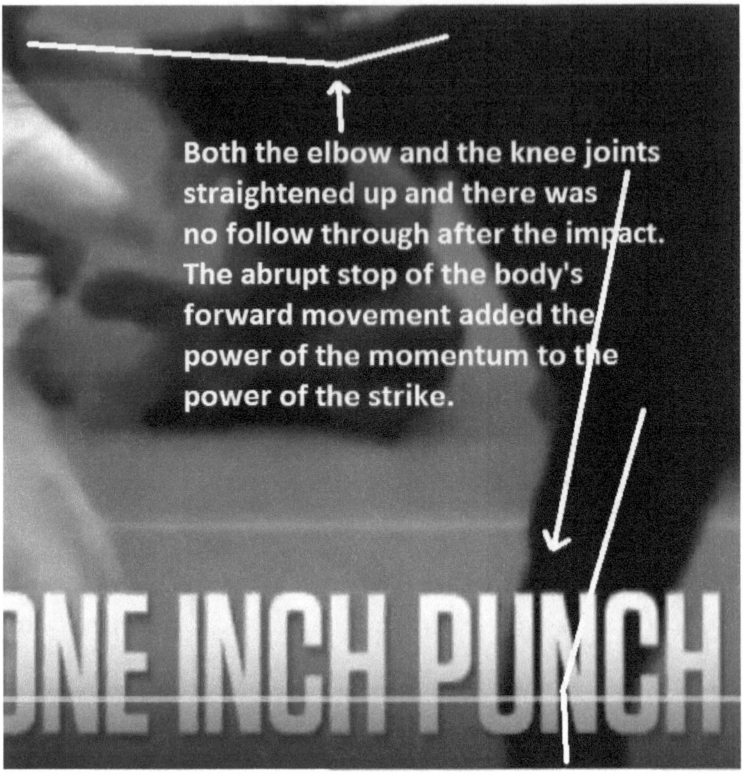

Both the elbow and the knee joints
straightened up and there was
no follow through after the impact.
The abrupt stop of the body's
forward movement added the
power of the momentum to the
power of the strike.

ONE INCH PUNCH

Subtitle: The Ji 擠 form of tai chi power explained and trained scientifically

Author: George Ho,

Coauthors: Jennifer Ho and Rebecca Ho

Copyright © 2019 George Ho,

All rights reserved.

This article covers many topics regarding this form of tai chi power. It is a part of my Med Rehab Tai Chi publication.

Some innovative topics in this booklet:

In this booklet, I have started with my scientific explanations of the mystical interpretation of the Ji form of tai chi power by a famous tai chi master, Master Wang Pui-sheng. Many people are impressed with tai chi masters' demonstrations of using this form of power to push demonstration partners flying up in the air. However, if this pushing technique can really be used in a real fight wouldn't it be used by highly paid sports professionals like Sumo wrestlers in Japan?

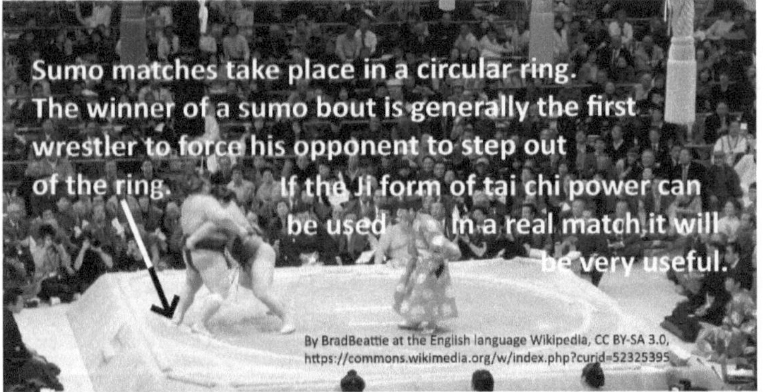

From my researches I have found that the origin of this powerful technique was discovered by Master 郭 Guo 雲深 yúnshēn (1829−1900) of 形意 xíng yì when he was handcuffed and shackled for three years in prison. 形意 xíng yì is a form of martial arts that stress heavily on pile stance training and footwork. Since Master Guo's movements were limited in prison, he could only practice pile stance and one step at time footwork. With a lot of practice, he created his 「Half step beng punch, 半(meaning half)步(meaning step)崩 (meaning collapse)拳(meaning fist); it is called bàn 半 bù 步 bēng 崩 quán 拳 in Chinese」, with which he knocked out many opponents in one punch. But his punch did not push people in the air. The tai chi demonstration of pushing people in the air was made famous by Yang 楊 shǎo hóu 少侯(1862-1930), one of the sons of Yang 楊 Lù chán 露禪, the founder of Yang style tai chi, who never bothered to demonstrate his real kung fu. Those newly conceived moves were his secret weapons that he wanted to be kept unknown to the public. As a bodyguard of the Qing's Imperial members, his kung fu was well witnessed when Yang 楊 Lù chán 露禪 protected his masters by hurting and even killing people. He was called 楊無敵 Yáng wúdí, the invincible Master Yang.

翁同龢 Wēng tónghé（1830－1904）

, a tutor of two Qing emperors composed a couplet to praise Yang's martial art skill:

「手捧太極震寰宇，胸懷絕技壓群雄

`Shǒu pěng tàijí zhèn huányǔ, xiōnghuái juéjì yā qúnxióng'」

My translation of the couplet: "With the taiji power in his hands and the well-concealed martial art moves he subdued all the heroes of the world"

I have a new theory why Yang 楊 Lù chán 露禪 and always won in a fight. I think he could sense the opponents' attacks from his premonitions, called "direct knowing"神通 Shéntōng in Buddhism. He might not be 100% accurate in his predictions but he had a rare and acquired advantage in any combat. A According to Master Sun Lutang 孫祿堂's 《拳意述真》 "172　　拳術至練虛合道，是將真意化到至虛至無之境，不動之時，內中寂然，空虛無一動其心，至於忽然有不測之事，雖不見不聞而能覺而避之。中庸云：「至誠之道可以前知」，是此意也。能到至誠之道者，三派拳術中，餘知有四人而已。形意拳李洛能先生，八卦拳董海川先生，太極拳楊露禪先生，武禹襄先生。四位先生皆有不見不聞之知覺。其餘諸先生，皆是見聞之知覺而已。如外不有測之事，只要眼見耳聞，無論來者如何疾快，俱能躲閃。因其功夫入於虛境而未到於至虛，不能有不見不聞之知覺也。其練他派拳術者，亦常聞有此境界，未能詳其姓氏，故未錄之。"

My translation:

 In the most advanced state martial arts is similar to Laozi's Daoism it is united to the universal Dao and therefore has the same miraculous quality to predict what is going to happen from some early signs. According to the Confucian Doctrine of the Mean, called 中庸, one of the Four Books in the Confucian Ethics, this manifestation of the advanced form of martial arts is referred to as, "至誠之道,可以前知…". It means that at the sophisticated level of one's religious or ethical belief one possesses the premonition to sense what is going to happen from forthcoming signs or premonitions that usually occur before an abrupt change of event. I (Sun) know that there are at least four martial arts masters, who possess this miraculous ability, Master 李洛能 Li Luoneng of Xingyiquan, Master 董海川 Dong Haichuan of Baqua quan, Master 楊露禪 Yang Luchen of Taijiquan.

After Master 楊露禪 Yang Luchen died his son, Yang 楊 shǎo hóu 少侯 did not get his job as a bodyguard. I think the main reason that he could not succeed his father's job was that he did not have his father's premonition skill and his ability as a bodyguard was in doubt. He could only make a living by teaching tai chi to the Qing's Imperial members and their friends.

I think this is why he thought of using the demonstration of bouncing partners flying up in the air to win his kung fu credibility. For fear of hurting his Imperial students, he trained Wang 汪 Yongquan 永泉 (1904-1987), an expert in Manchurian wrestling as his demonstration partner because just like judo a skillful Manchuria wrestler is not afraid of falling.

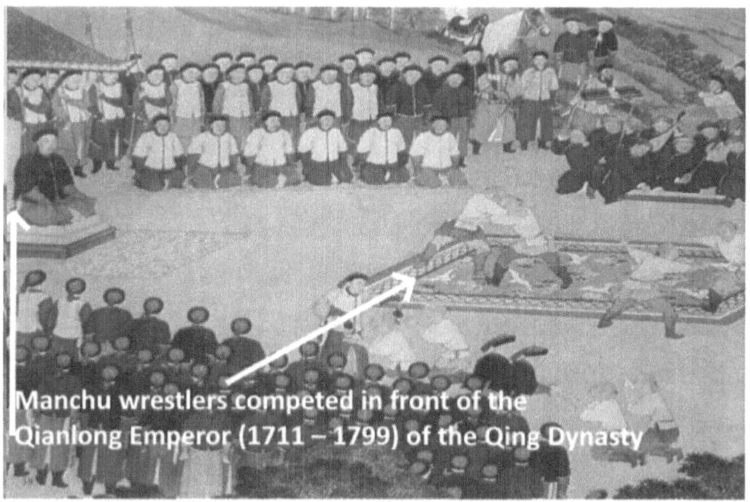

Manchu wrestlers competed in front of the Qianlong Emperor (1711 – 1799) of the Qing Dynasty

As a demonstration partner Wang had to be fully instructed in how to add the momentum force of his running towards the demonstration master in order to enhance the power that sent him flying up in the air. This is why Wang could learn this special kung fu that was regarded as a family secret of Yang style tai chi.

Then came Bruce Lee, who was a kung fu fanatic and he probably read about all the above people and their skills in martial art. His one-inch punch and six-inch punch are just as effective as the Ji form of tai chi power. The mechanics are very similar. However, his martial arts training did not help his epilepsy, which is a common brain disorder characterized by recurrent seizures. Again from my researches, I think he did not practice his static meditation in a way so that he could do Liàn jīng huà qì,

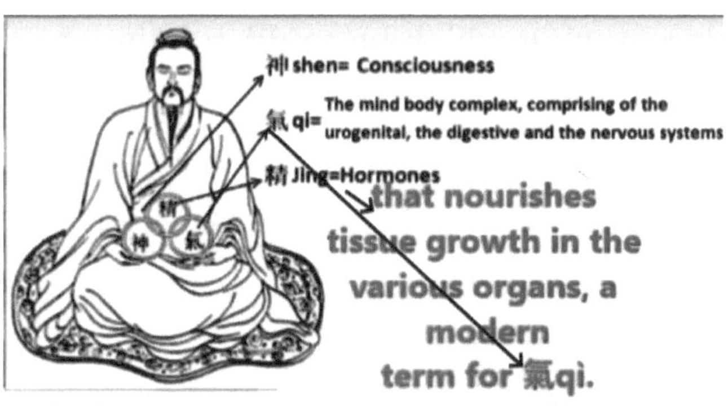

the process in which jīng (hormonal secretion is my scientific conception of jing 精) is used to stimulate the further development of the nervous system, vaguely called qi in Chinese. Please read his famous quote about meditation,

"Be like water making its way through cracks." Please compare Bruce's conception of meditation with the highly sophisticated Buddhist meditation method, called 6 Wonderful Ways, 六妙法門 Liù miàofǎ mén, that could lead to 禪定 chán ding, in which one can enhance one's wisdom, the sign of the evolution of the nervous system. With his highly sophisticated martial arts as a form of Dong gong he could probably cure his epilepsy with a good Jing gong practice of static meditation, during which he could acquire the essential breathing technique, called 報身氣 Bào shēn qì in Buddhism or 胎息 Taixi, the Embryonic mode of respiration in Daoism.

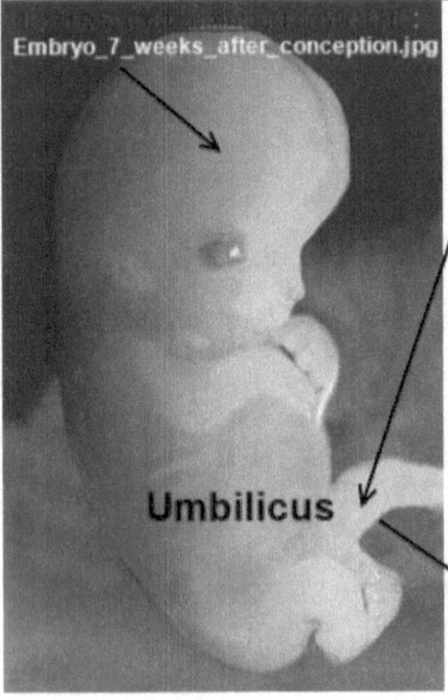

Breathing is the process of moving air into and out of the lungs to facilitate gas exchange with the internal environment, mostly by bringing in oxygen and flushing out carbon dioxide.

In physiology, **respiration** is defined as the movement of oxygen from the outside environment to the cells within tissues, and the transport of carbon dioxide in the opposite direction. You could also define respiration as **the release of energy from glucose** and this is achieved through the breaking down of this glucose in the cells and oxygen from the atmosphere is absolutely pivotal to this breaking down.

In Chinese both Breathing and respiration are called 呼吸 Hūxī.

The illustrations in the picture have been enlarged:

—

Breathing is the process of moving air into and out of the lungs to facilitate gas exchange with the internal environment, mostly by bringing in oxygen and flushing out carbon dioxide.

In physiology, **respiration** is defined as the movement of oxygen from the outside environment to the cells within tissues, and the transport of carbon dioxide in the opposite direction. You could also define respiration as **the release of energy from glucose** and this is achieved through the breaking down of this glucose in the cells and oxygen from the atmosphere is absolutely pivotal to this breaking down.

In Chinese both Breathing and respiration are called 呼吸 Hūxī.

Master Sun Lutang, who demonstrated Master

15 dong jin

Guo's 「Half step beng punch」in this booklet
is the best example of how to complement his
martial arts training as a form of Dong gong
with his pile stance as a form of Jing gong and
he attained Enlightenment. Master 郭 Guo 雲深

yúnshēn's 「Half step beng punch」also shows
us that the form of dong gong that complements
jing gong does not have to be complicated or
slow like tai chi quan as a form of martial arts.
I have experimented with walking, swimming
and using the various tennis strokes as the
different levels of dong gong practice and initial
results are encouraging.

6 Wonderful Ways, 六妙法門 Liù miàofǎ mén:

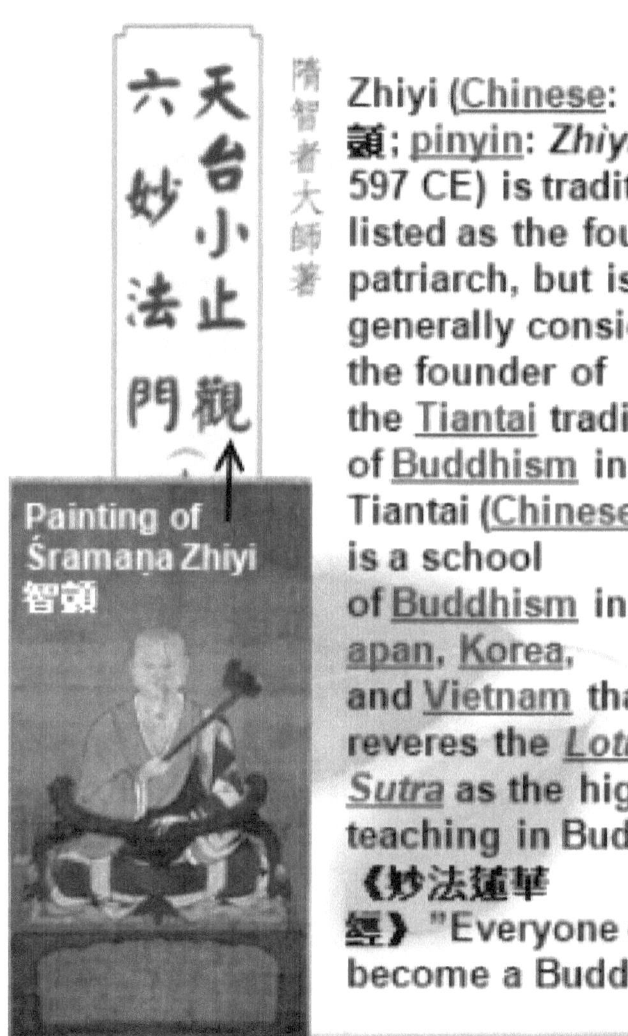

Zhiyi (Chinese: 智顗; pinyin: *Zhiyi*;, (538–597 CE) is traditionally listed as the fourth patriarch, but is generally considered the founder of the Tiantai tradition of Buddhism in China. Tiantai (Chinese: 天台;) is a school of Buddhism in China, Japan, Korea, and Vietnam that reveres the *Lotus Sutra* as the highest teaching in Buddhism 《妙法蓮華經》 "Everyone can become a Buddha.

According to Master Nan:止(breath cessation)為(is)定(*Samatha's*)之母(mother)、定為(is)止之果(result)。觀(meditation)為(is)慧(wisdom's)之母(mother)、慧為(is)觀之果。6妙門(6 wonderful ways)中前三步(the first 3 ways)，1/數(counting the breath)、2/隨(follow 止)、3/止屬於定學(for *Samatha*)。後三步(the last 3 ways)，4/觀、5/還(return to 法身"truth body")、6/淨(Purity)，則屬於慧學領域。

Disclaimer:

This article has been written with extensive researches. However, all the suggestions and recommendations are meant to be educational and are not intended to be a substitute for customized advice from your personal doctor or health professional. The author will not be liable to any loss, injury, or damage allegedly arising from any information or suggestion in this book.

Preface

In the last century we have witnessed a global acceptance of Western medicine as the healthcare mainstream because of its progress and reliability through scientific research. However, history has shown us that prolonged power domination usually leads to oligarchical developments. Western pharmaceutical companies are concrete examples of this historical pattern. They have developed many patented ways of controlling chronic illnesses instead of curing them. Cheaper treatment methods that cannot be patented are put aside and even suppressed because they cannot be turned into profit. Movies like "The Cocoon" have shown to the world that many seniors are not living but just existing with the help of these medications. Many of them are dreaming of regaining their health or just dying gracefully. Some social groups have even advocated euthanasia, which will become problematic when practiced on a large scale with cumbersome legislative control. This solution is too artificial, relying too much on the government's regulation of something that is highly personal.

Medical-Rehab-Tai-Chi (MRTC) has extracted wisdom of past and contemporary sages in regaining health through lifestyle changes. Dr. Ho has researched extensively to medically substantiate the health practices of Tai Chi, Zen meditation, yoga and Qigong etc.

Some harmful ancient ways of training like the low stance in Tai Chi has been examined from a medical perspective and modified scientifically to make it safe and efficient. Some unscientific claims made by some health groups were examined and rebutted with known scientific knowledge. Hopefully MRTC can be scientifically developed so that it can help people live a relatively drug-free and control-free life and die peacefully with dignity without troubling anyone. If many people can do so the medical cost shouldered by the baby boomers and their offspring will be solved easily, not by the government but by the people themselves.

Contents:

1.My scientific explanation of the Master Pui-sheng Wang's unions of acupuncture points to power the Ji form of power is that they are symbolic expressions of the unique nature of the tai chi adhesive footwork, which is controlled by the Dantian that forms the abdominal part of the CranioSacral postural reflex of tai chi. I have a YouTube movie that briefly introduces my self-published article: p.24

2. How to practice the Ji form of power: p.40

3.Using a concrete example to show the training of the Ji form of tai chi power…p.64

4.The demonstration of the explosive Ji power as shown in the above picture probably originated from the demonstrations by Yang 楊 shǎo hóu 少侯…p.73

5.To have the privilege of inheriting the Yang style kung fu secret Wang 汪 Yongquan 永泉

1. My scientific explanation of the Master Pui-sheng Wang's unions of acupuncture points to power the Ji form of power is that they are symbolic expressions of the unique nature of the tai chi adhesive footwork, which is controlled by the Dantian that forms the abdominal part of the CranioSacral postural reflex of tai chi. I have a YouTube movie that briefly introduces my self-published article:

The Ji 擠 form of tai chi power is often used by many famous masters in demonstrations to throw people up in the air as seen in the YouTube video, 鄭曼青 - 推手 (A Yang style master, *Zhèng Mànqīng – push hand*; the link is below:

https://www.youtube.com/watch?v=eTOEjBWFr-8
鄭曼青 - 推手 **The push-hand part is at 2.37.**

For a more dramatic demonstration by Master Frantzis shown on his book cover please Google:

- **The Power of Internal Martial Arts and Chi: Combat and Energy Secrets of Ba Gua, Tai Chi and Hsing-I by**

- <u>Bruce Frantzis</u>

The link show of the cover of this book is <u>http://www.barnesandnoble.com/w/the-power-of-internal-martial-arts-and-chi-bruce-frantzis/1111615333?ean=9781583941904</u>

In my three decades of being a chiropractor and a tai chi practitioner I have seen a lot of injuries from the practice and demonstrations of tai chi push hand. In this article I have demonstrated better and more effective ways to train and evaluate one's tai chi power than to throw people around in order to train for tai chi power.

The following mystical explanations of the Ji form of tai chi power is by Master Wang Pui-sheng. I am supplementing his theories with my scientific explanations:

Wang Peisheng (1919–2004) was a teacher of Wu-style t'ai chi ch'uan. He was Yang Yuting's student and also a student of Wang Mao Zhai.

He began training in martial arts with the Baguazhang master Ma Gui learning Yin Style Ba Gua Zhang 64 Palms. He assisted Yang Yu Ting teaching t'ai chi from the age of 15. He became the head of the Northern Wu-style t'ai chi ch'uan group in Beijing after the death of Yang Yu Ting in 1982.

Although most famous for his taijiquan he began his long career by studying Yin baguazhang with the 3rd generation master Ma Gui. He was also very good at tongbeiquan, tantui, xingyiquan, and bajiquan, having studied with famous masters of each of these arts.

https://en.wikipedia.org/wiki/Wang_Peisheng

According to Master Wáng 王 péishēng 培生's mystical acupunctural and I Jing (the Book of Change) explanations the explosive power of the 擠 ji is because of the summation of 2 unions of 2 sets of Earthly Branches represented by 2 sets of acupuncture points. Master Wang's instruction for the 1ˢᵗ union of those points is "The rear foot looks for the front foot." Master Wang inferred this from the solid bottom stroke of the trigram, 震 Zhèn☳, which is like an upright pot. In the diagram below the left foot's acupuncture point 湧泉穴 (yǒng quán xué) is Earth Branch 3, the yin 寅 Earth

Branch and the right 湧泉 is 12, the hai 亥 Earth Branch.

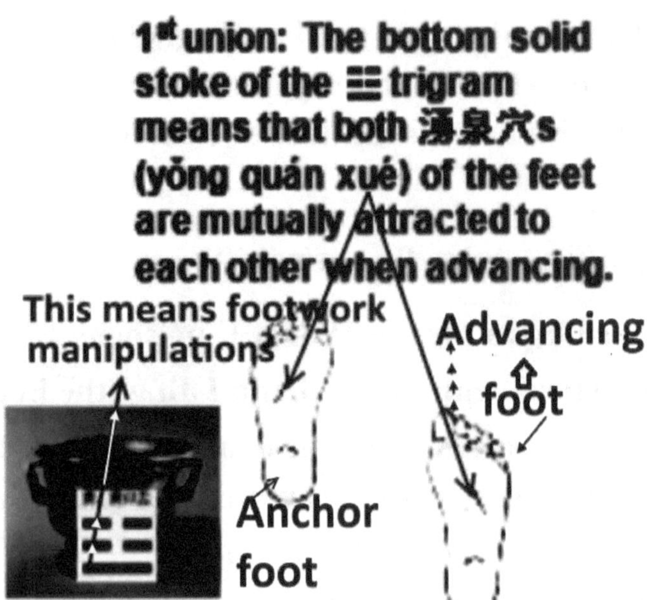

The author of this article, Dr. Ho's scientific explanations of Master Wang symbolic I Jing descriptions of the Ji form of tai chi power:

One of the forces of the Ji power is generated by the momentum or impetus of the body when the body is pushed forward by the advancing foot, symbolically described by Master Wang as the union of the two Yong quan xues or as the union of the 3rd and the 4th Earth Branches, shown below.

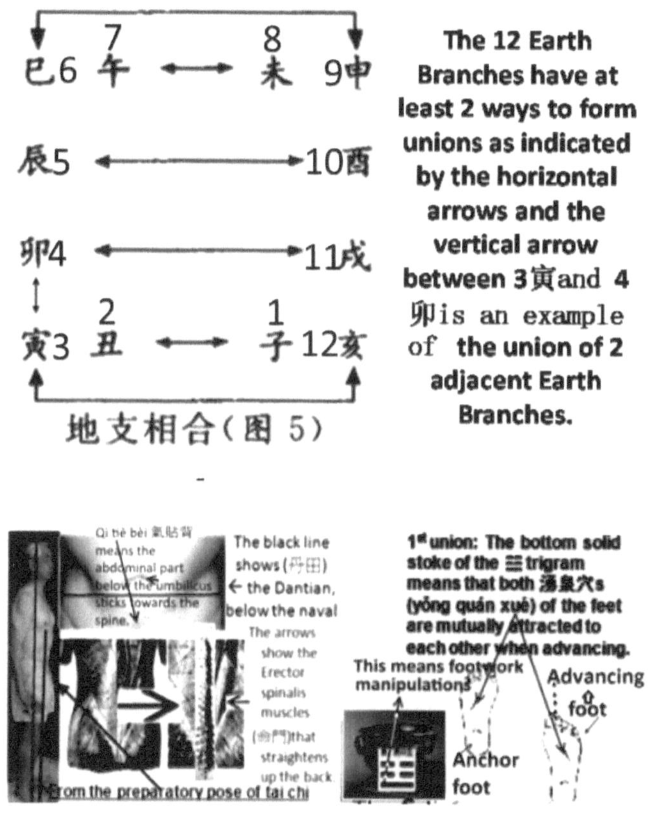

Two bigger pictures are shown below when the above picture is divided into 2 parts:

The conditions that form the 1st union is that you have to have the CranioSacral postural reflex of tai chi before the union of the two acupuncture points (yong quan xue) footwork shown in the 2nd picture can have internal power of one's tai chi kung fu:

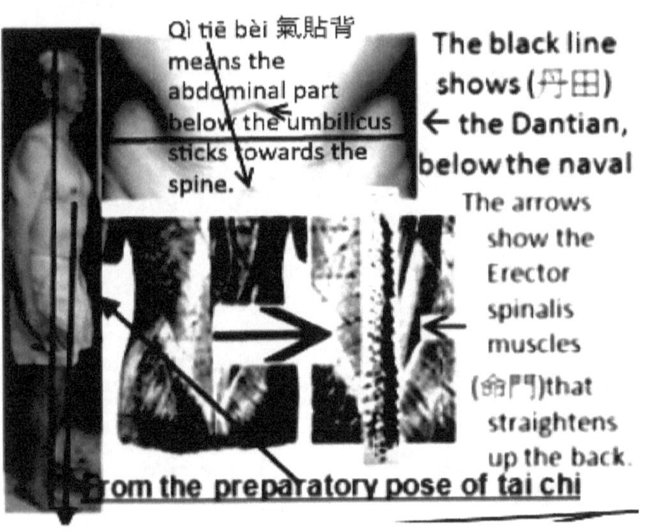

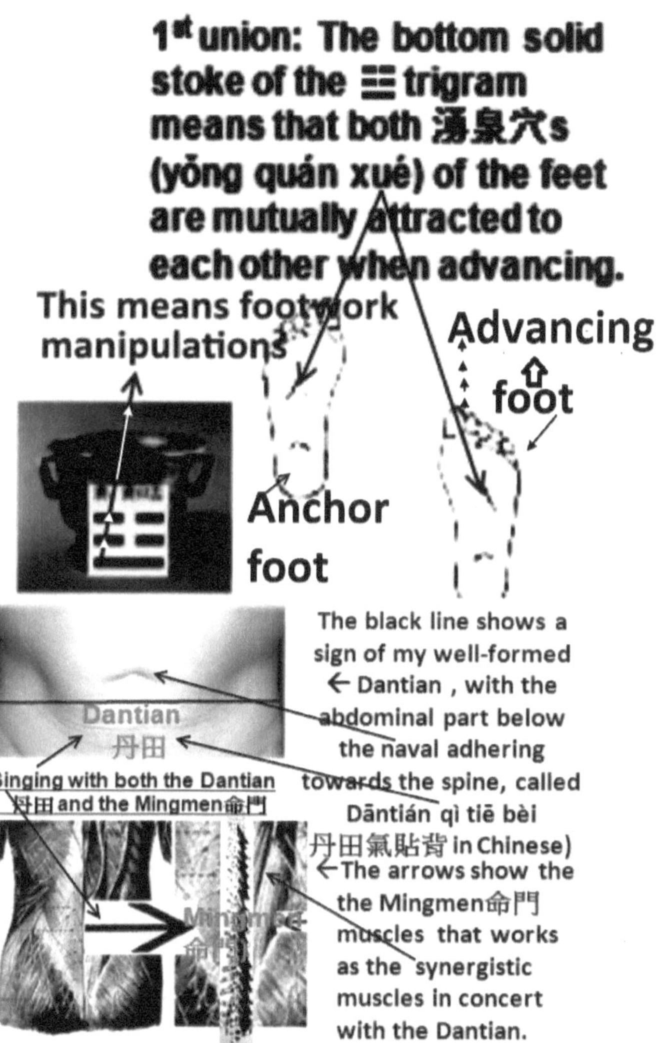

The concrete conditions of the CranioSacral postural reflex of tai chi are:

Qi Tie Bei= The abdominal part below the umbilicus sticks towards the spine, as shown in the pictures above and

Ding Tou Xuan= The head feels so light as if it was hanging in the air by a hook, as shown in the picture below:

The <u>**Tai Chi CranioSacral Postural Reflex**</u> **that fosters** <u>Tai Chi Kung Fu for Back and Health Enhancement</u>

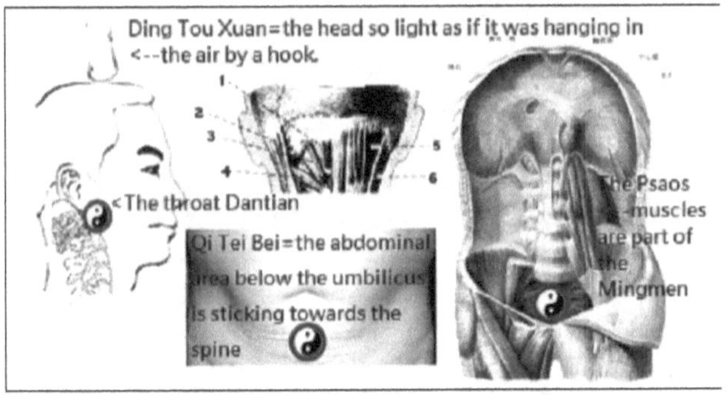

The purpose of doing Tai Chi is to acquire a unique postural reflex that makes you feel the head as light as if it was hanging from a hook. This postural reflex can be acquired by practicing tai chi and or meditation.

By: Dr. George Ho, B. Soc. Sc., M.A., D.C.

Coauthors: Jennifer Ho and Rebecca Ho

As shown in the picture below, the body is pushed forward by the advancing rear foot while the front foot anchors the body waiting for the advancing rear foot. The union of the two feet creates the impetus because the advance of the whole body stops at the anchor foot.

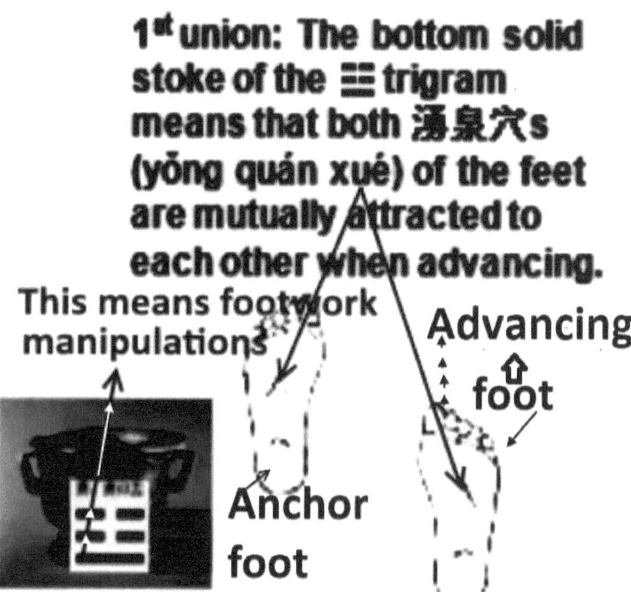

The above picture helps explain the formation of the first force of the two combined forces of the Ji form of tai chi power according to Master Wang. It is from the momentum of the push of the pusher with the internal kung fu from the abdominal Dantian and the Mingmen the force is suddenly stopped at the upper-back level, where the acupuncture point, Jia ji xue is at the 4th Earth Branch in the picture below.

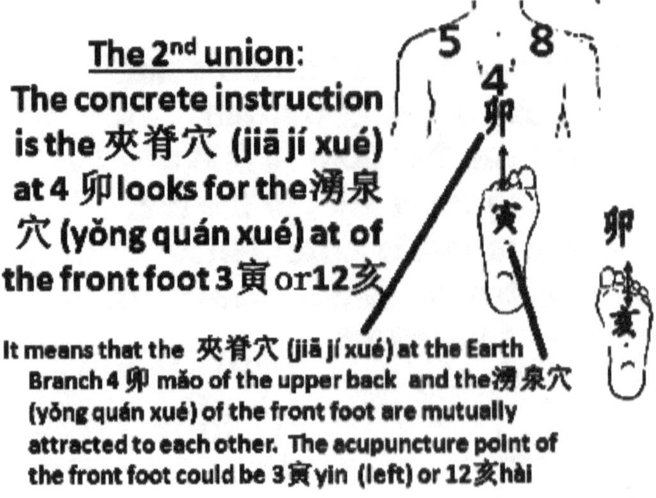

If you have a good Dantian supported by the Mingmen you can feel the extra strength from that level physically when you strike at anything and vocally when you sing or speak.

Listening to one's singing or chanting is an easy way to evaluate his or her Dantian. If you ask any Chinese opera fan, he or she can tell you which singers have strong Dantian just from listening to their singing or even speaking. I have been told that I have a good Dantian. You can listen to my singing on YouTube or my narrations on my YouTube movies and hear for yourself.

The 2nd acupunctural meridian union that forms the Ji form of power according to Master Wáng 王 péishēng 培生's mystical acupunctural and I Jing (the Book of Change) explanations is explained by the following instructions. Please refer to the diagram below:

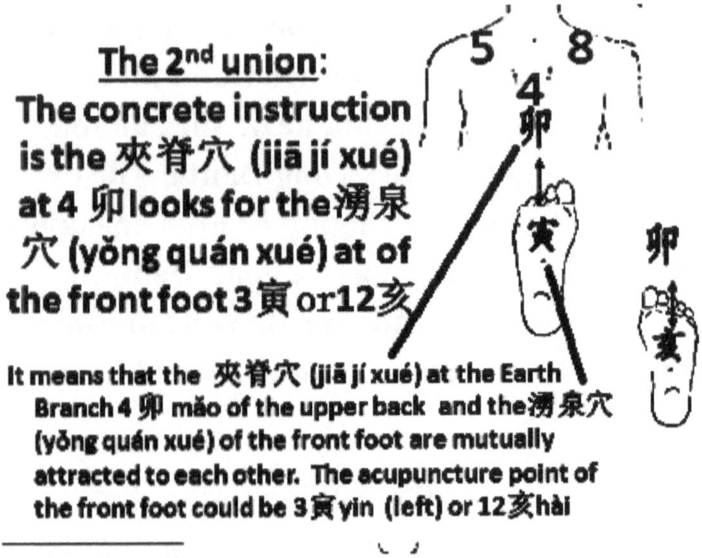

The concrete instruction of the 2nd union by Master Wang is that the 夾脊穴 (jiā jí xué) at 4 卯 looks for the 湧泉穴 (yǒng quán xué) at of the front foot 3 寅 or 12 亥. It means that the 夾脊穴 (jiā jí xué) at the Earth Branch 4 卯 mǎo of the upper back and the 湧泉穴 (yǒng quán xué) of the front foot are mutually attracted to each other. The acupuncture point of the front foot could be 3 寅 yin (left) or 12 亥 hài (right) . The 12 Earth Branches have at least 2 ways to form unions as indicated by the horizontal arrows and the vertical arrow between 3 寅 and

4 卯 is an example of the union of 2 adjacent Earth Branches.

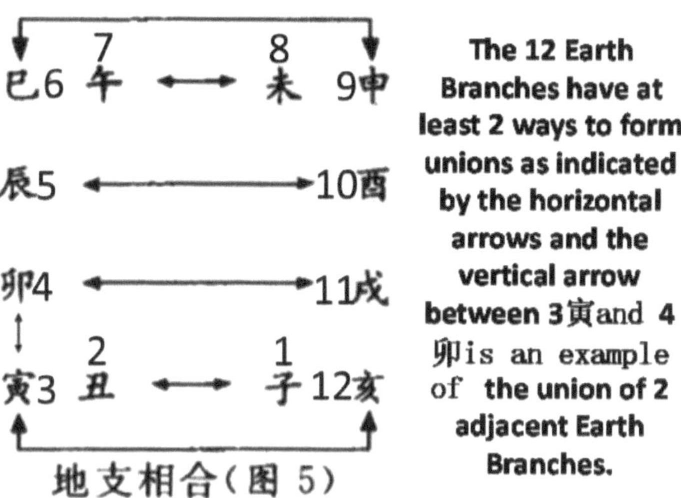

地支相合（图 5）

The 12 Earth Branches have at least 2 ways to form unions as indicated by the horizontal arrows and the vertical arrow between 3寅and 4 卯is an example of the union of 2 adjacent Earth Branches.

The mystical terms are explained with the pictures shown below:

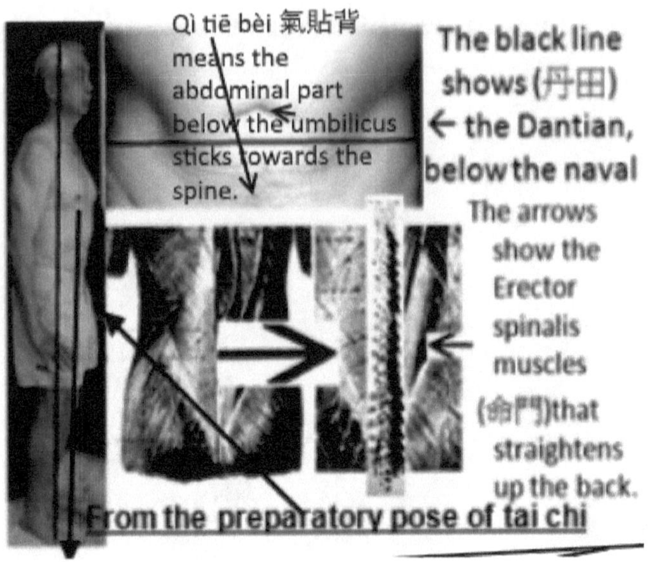

   The first condition of this 2nd union is again you have to have the CranioSacral postural reflex with a good Dantian. The second condition of the 2nd union is that the front foot has to anchor at the vertical line of the 夾脊穴 (jiā jí xué) acupuncture point at the upper-back.

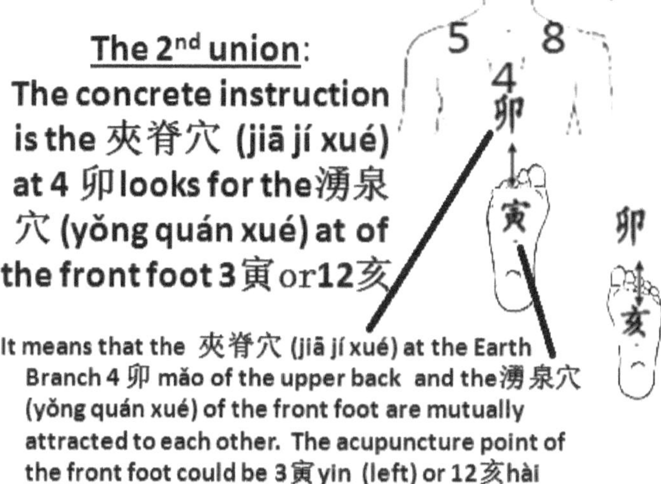

My modern explanation of the formation of this part of the Ji form of tai chi power as shown in the above picture:

The formation of the above acupunctural point union is just a symbolic expression of a sudden and abrupt stop of the body's rapid forward advancement in order to use the forward momentum to enhance the power of impact on the oncoming opponent.

2.How to practice the Ji form of power:

a. Assume the preparatory pose of tai chi that has the acquired CranioSacral Postural reflex as shown below:

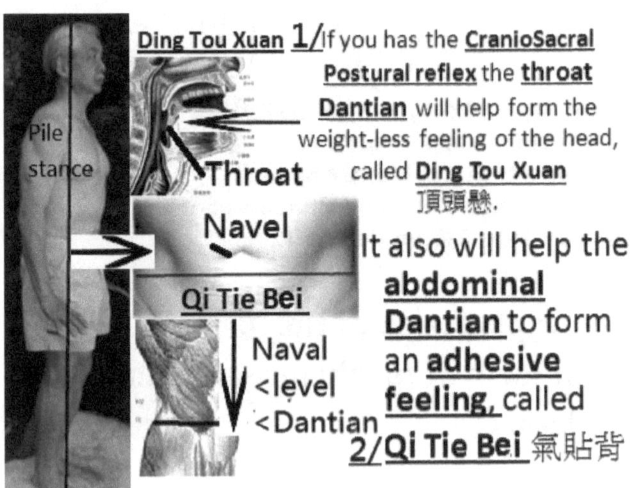

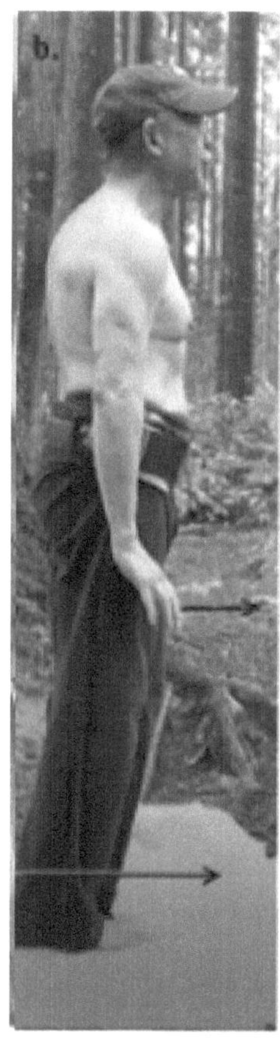

b. Get ready to raise the arms with the Peng form of power by manipulating the CranioSacral Postural reflex, shown in the picture above.
If you just raise your arms with the muscles attached to the arms and shouldes you are not practicing tai chi because there is no Peng power, controlled by the CranioSacral Postural reflex.

Get ready to raise the arms with the Peng form of power by manipulating the CranioSacral Postural reflex. If you just raise your arms with the muscles attached to the arms you are not practicing tai chi because there is no Peng power, controlled by the CranioSacral Postural reflex.

The comparison of just (a) slowly raising the arms with the shoulder muscles with (b) raising the arms with the Peng form of tai chi power is like walking (a) and bicycle riding (b).

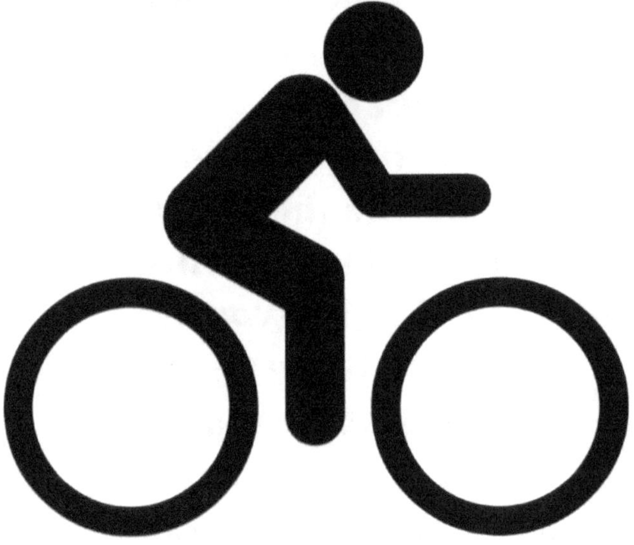

The two sets of movements are governed by two different sets of reflexes. Many people think that tai chi is just moving slowly and smoothly. Practicing tai chi like this without acquiring a new set of reflexes will never give you any significant health benefits and it is useless in self-defence. However, once you have acquired the CranioSacral Postural reflex you can apply it in any posture and any kind of movements, fast like playing tennis or slow like walking and swimming.

When you are learning to acquire the CranioSacral Postural reflex, you do tai chi slowly. It is like learning how to ride a bicycle on an easy-to-ride bicycle and once you have learned the reflex you want to ride a more difficult to maneuver bicycle to train for strengthening the muscles and the reflex.

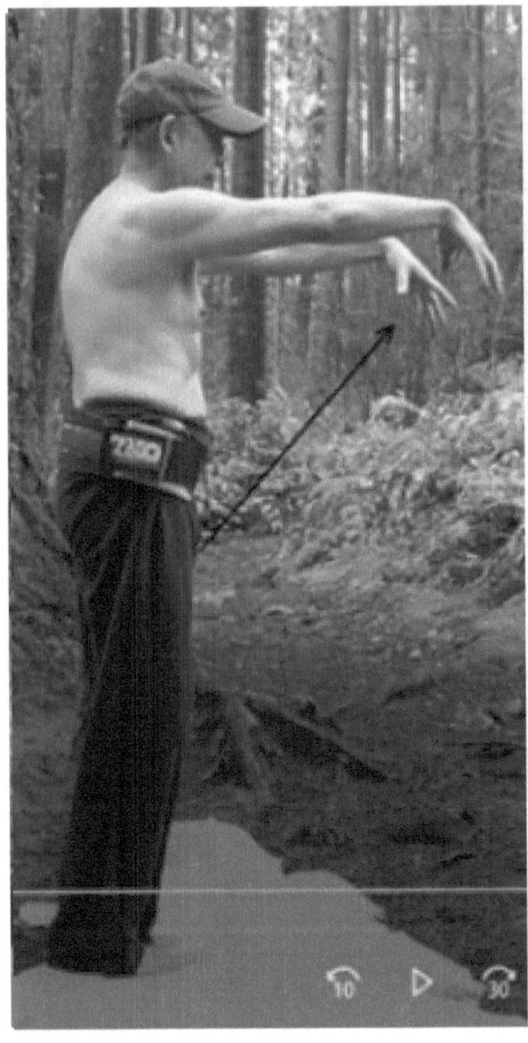

c. Raise the arms with the Peng form of power.

44 dong jin

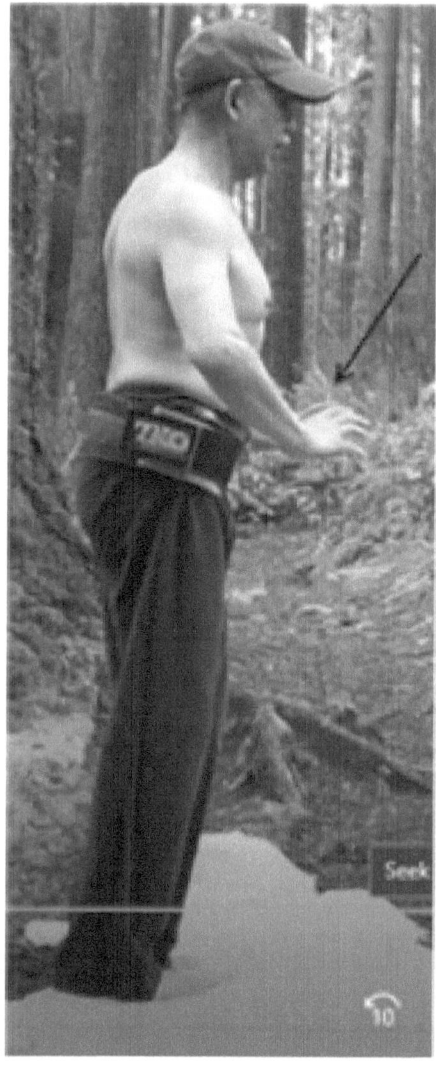

d.
Lower
the
arms
with
the An
form of
power.

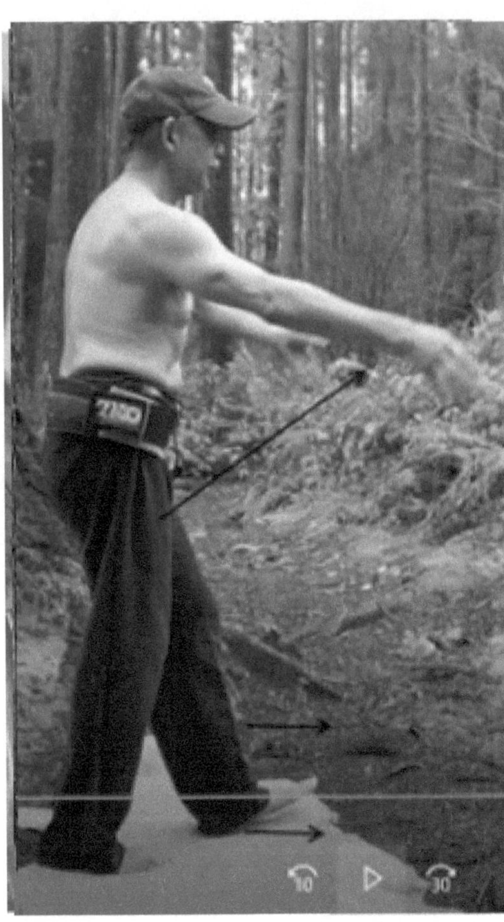

e. Raise the arms with the Peng form of power and take one step forward simultaneously.

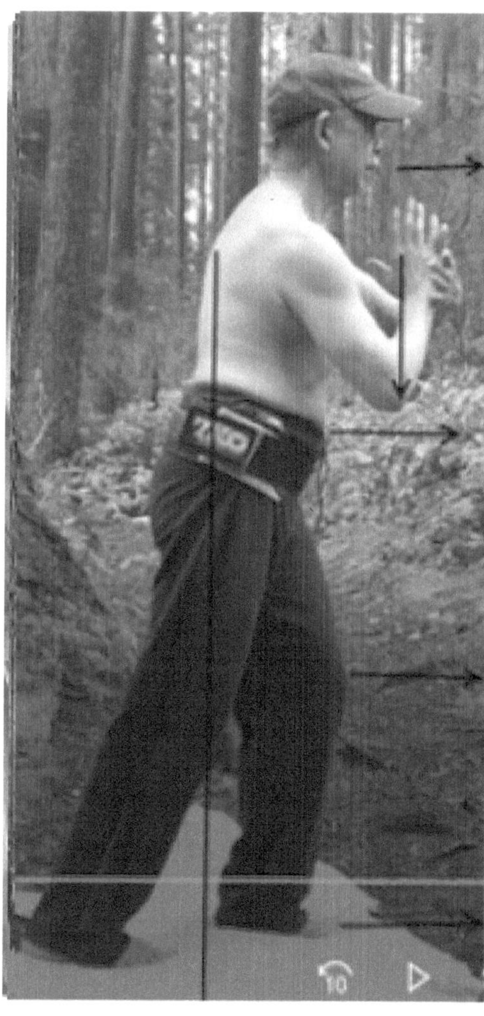

f. Form the arms to get ready for doing the Ji form of power.

47 dong jin

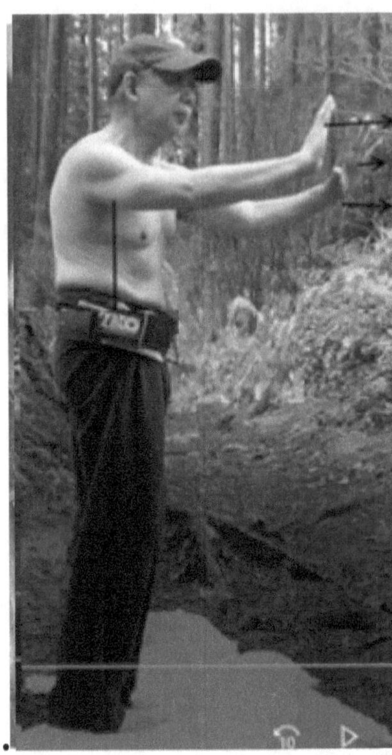

g.
Execute the Ji form of tai chi power with the advancing rear foot (the right one here) joining the anchor foot (left) with a push of the hands.
These 2 forces are further reinforced by the Dantian force from the lower abdomen

48 dong jin

There is a YouTube movie demonstrating the above movements of the Peng, An, Ji and Lu forms of tai chi power. This is the link:

https://www.youtube.com/watch?v=YdvrmvHA0ow&list=PL9RRMUY60ixTdZpWGySNpmYtCPSmegRpk&index=15

Singing the Silent Night as background music for doing the 4 forms of tai chi power by Dr. George Ho

Master Wang's unions of acupuncture points to power the Ji form of power is that they are symbolic expressions of the unique characteristic of the tai chi adhesive footwork, which is controlled by the Dantian that forms the abdominal part of the CranioSacral postural reflex of tai chi. I have a YouTube movie that briefly introduces my Kindle book: Acquiring the CranioSacral Postural Reflex with Meditation and Tai Chi for Longevity and Enlightenment (Tai chi and meditation Book 12)

https://www.amazon.com/dp/B07NCBN3DX

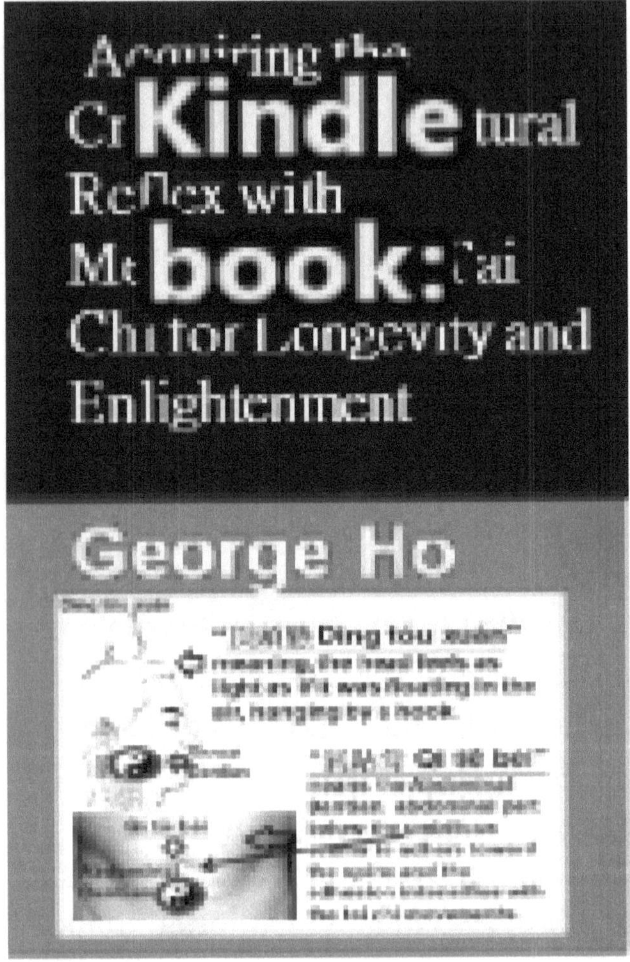

A clear picture is shown below:

50 dong jin

The <u>Tai Chi CranioSacral Postural Reflex</u> that fosters <u>Tai Chi Kung Fu for Back and Health Enhancement</u>

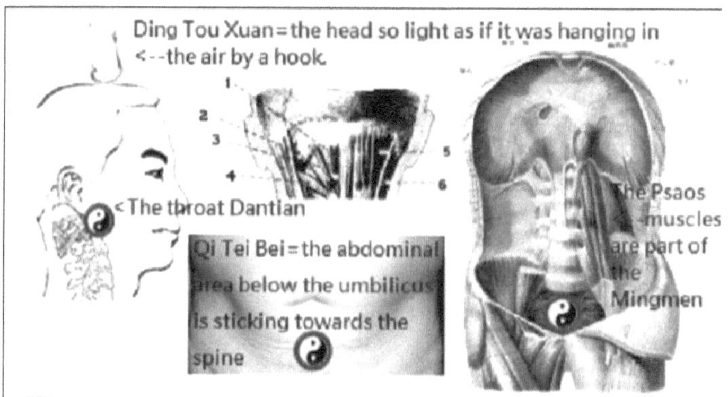

The purpose of doing Tai Chi is to acquire a unique postural reflex that makes you feel the head as light as if it was hanging from a hook. This postural reflex can be acquired by practicing tai chi and or meditation.

By: Dr. George Ho, B. Soc. Sc., M.A., D.C.

I also have an article, called "Going Beyond the Term Relaxation" published in the 2014 Spring

51 dong jin

edition of T'ai Chi magazine. In that article I used two signs mentioned in the tai chi classics to coin the new postural concept, the

Tai Chi CranioSacral Postural Reflex:

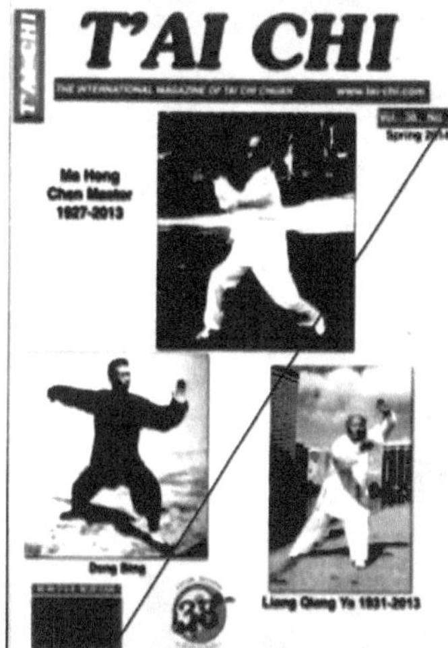

My article in the 2014 Spring issue of T'ai Chi Magazine

The Importance of the CranioSacral postural reflex in Tai Chi by Dr. George Ho, B.Soc. Sc.,M.A.,D.C.

"鬆開 Song kai" was one of the key principles in Tai Chi that was heavily emphasized by Master Chengfu Yang 楊澄甫 (1883-1936), the 3rd generation representative of Yang style Tai Chi. He emphasized that in practice as well as in real combats the whole body has to be in a "鬆開 Song kai" state. Otherwise one will be forced into the defensive and reactive status all the time.

One of his students, Master Man-ching Cheng 鄭 曼青（1902－1975）was the 4th generation representative of Yang style Tai Chi. He said it took him 50 years to really experience what his teacher, Master Chengfu Yang 楊澄甫 meant by "鬆開 Song kai", translated by鄭Cheng's team of students as a state of "relaxation". 曼青蜜所飲述：「鬆所每日必重言十餘次，要鬆要鬆；要鬆淨，要全身鬆開，反之則日不鬆、不鬆、不鬆就是挨打的架子。」(鄭)

One of Master Man-ching Cheng students, Mr. Benjamin Lo (Luóbāngzhēn羅邦楨, 1925-) of San Francisco was asked in an interview in 2001 regarding the main principles of Tai Chi. He maintained that "relaxation" was the most important one and when he was asked how to become relaxed he said doing the Tai Chi forms was the only way he knew. He said doing the forms would lead to the posture to acquire this elusive state of "relaxation".

6

The Importance of the CranioSacral postural reflex in Tai Chi by
Dr. George Ho, B.Soc. Sc.,M.A.,D.C.

"鬆開 Song kai" was one of the key principles in Tai Chi that was heavily emphasized by Master Chengfu Yang 楊澄甫 (1883-1936), the 3rd generation representative of Yang style Tai Chi. He emphasized that in practice as well as in real combats the whole body has to be in a "鬆開 Song kai" state. Otherwise one will be forced into the defensive and reactive status all the time.

One of his students, Master Man-ching Cheng 鄭曼青（1902－1975）was the 4th generation representative of Yang style Tai Chi. He said it took him 50 years to really experience what his teacher, Master Chengfu Yang 楊澄甫 meant by "鬆開 Song kai", translated by 鄭 Cheng's team of students as a state of "relaxation". 曼青宗師說過：「澄師每日必要言十幾次，要鬆要鬆；要鬆淨，要全身鬆開。反之則曰不鬆、不鬆，不鬆就是挨打的架子。」(鄭)

One of Master Man-ching Cheng students, Mr. Benjamin Lo (Luóbāngzhèn 羅邦楨, 1925-   ) of San Francisco was asked in an interview in 2001 regarding the main principles of Tai Chi. He maintained that "relaxation" was the most important one and when he was asked how to become relaxed he said doing the Tai Chi forms was the only way he knew. He said doing the forms would lead to the posture to acquire this elusive state of "relaxation".

6

54 dong jin

The link of the YouTube movie that introduces this Kindle book is:

https://www.youtube.com/watch?v=mCOrxQw7pa4&t=26s

2 crucial concepts of tai chi, called dǒng jìn 懂勁 and 弸勁 péng jìn published in T'ai Chi Magazine

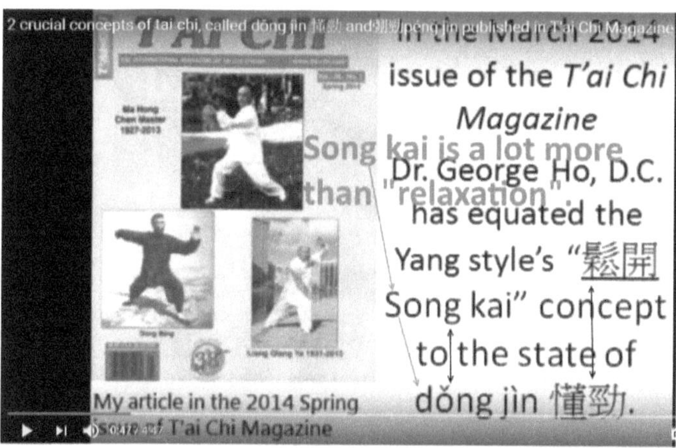

I have enriched this article into a Kindle book:

The Correct Interpretations of Two Important Tai Chi Concepts: "鬆開 Song kai" by Yang Chengfu 楊澄甫 and Peng jin 弸勁, the Peng form of concentrated Tai Chi ... of Taiji (Tai Chi and meditation Book 10)

https://www.amazon.com/dp/B07J2SC4KV

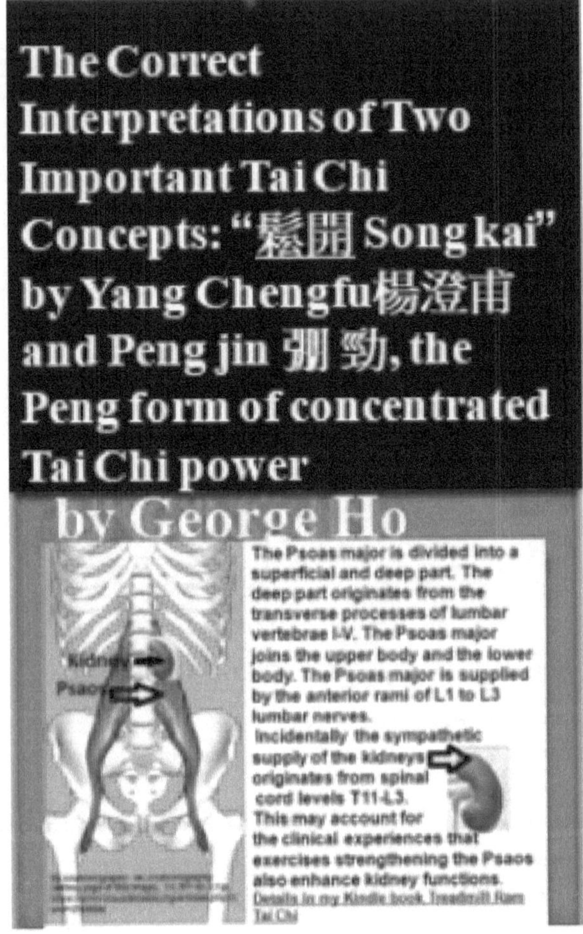

I have also published an ebook on Amazon.ca; "The Benefits of tai chi for the spine: The postural enhancement effect of tai chi, called the CranioSacral Postural reflex of Tai Chi (Tai chi and meditation Book 2)"

https://www.amazon.com/dp/B07D8GVFCY

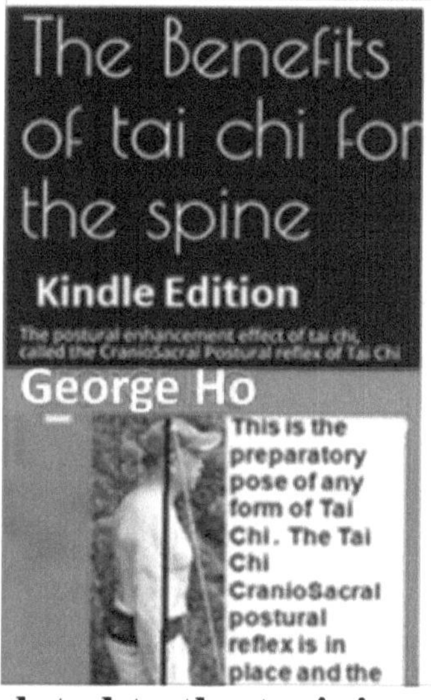

Related to the training of all the 8 forms of tai chi power, including the Ji form is Master 楊澄甫 (1883–1936, the 3rd generation gatekeeper of Yang's tai chi) Yang Chengfu's concept of "鬆開 Song kai". There are a lot of misinterpretations of "鬆開 Song kai", which has been misleadingly translated as "relaxation". "鬆開 Song kai" is a lot more than "relaxation". When you have reached the state of "懂勁 dong jin" according to the tai chi classics then you can really know what Master Yang Cheng-fu meant by "Song kai".

Dǒng 懂 in Chinese literally means to know and jìn 勁 means strength. Dǒng jìn can be better visualized in the aforementioned concrete expressions of "storing up power like a bow being drawn and release it like a heavily loaded arrow 蓄勁如張弓，發勁如放箭", according to Yǔxiāng Wǔ's (1812-1880) 武禹襄.

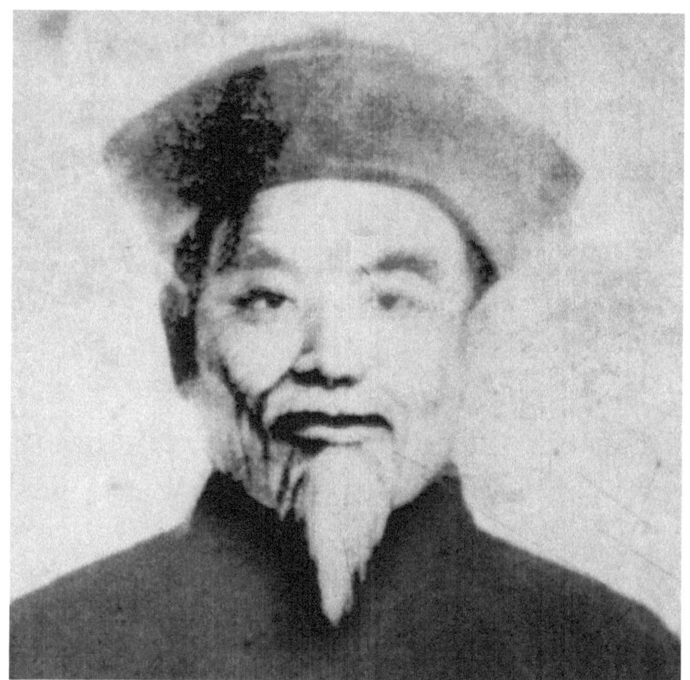

A picture of Wǔyǔxiāng 武禹襄

This is the goal of your practice in the 著熟 (Zhe shú) state, which is the reason why the movements are done slowly so that you can practice "loading the body with power" like a drawn bow and releasing the power like an arrow. When the 著熟 (Zhe shú) is sophisticated "Song kai" will occur naturally.

After reaching this state of dǒng jìn one's Tai Chi kung fu can improve qualitatively by the continuous practice of the complementary cooperative actions of the yin and the yang. The more one practices the better the Tai Chi dǒng jìn kung fu will become. The original text of the above translation is as followed, "陰 陽 相濟方 為懂勁。懂勁後。愈練愈精。" (陰 =yin, 陽 =yang, 相濟= complementing each other, 方為 懂勁。懂勁後=after the acquisition of dong jin。愈練愈精=continuous improvement。

蓄勁 Xù jìn 如張弓(a drawn bow)，發勁 fā jìn 如放箭(a shooting arrow).

蓄勁 Xù jìn represents the 陰 =yin, the power storing state like a bow being drawn and 發勁 fā jìn represents the 陽=yang state like a shooting arrow. When they can 相濟= complement each other, you have reached the 方為懂勁 (dong jin) state. This is the goal and the principle when you practice your tai chi movements.

One of his students, Master Man-ching Cheng 鄭 (鄭 has been translated as Cheng and

Zheng) 曼青（1902－1975）was the 4th generation representative of Yang style Tai Chi. He wrote in his book, *Zheng Zi tai chi chuan thirteen articles*

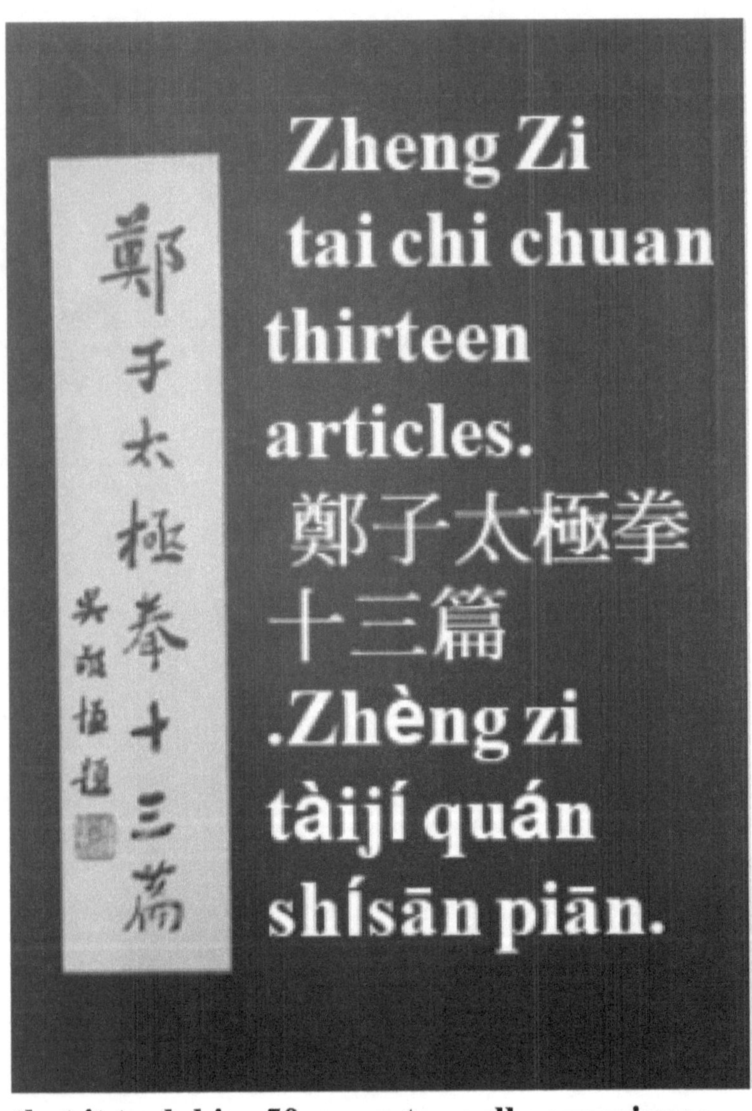

that it took him 50 years to really experience
what his teacher, Master Chengfu Yang 楊澄甫

meant by "鬆開 Song kai", translated by 鄭 Cheng's team of students as a state of "relaxation". 曼青宗師敘述：「澄師每日必重言十餘次，要鬆要鬆；要鬆淨，要全身鬆開。反之則曰不鬆、不鬆。不鬆就是挨打的架子。」[i](鄭. P.53)

3. Using a concrete example to show the training of the Ji form of tai chi power:

I shall use some pictures captured from a 1972 movie showing the training of the Ji form of power by a student of Zhèng Mànqīng, who was the representative of the 4th generation Yang style tai chi.

The following link of the movie is the one that the following pictures were captured:

https://www.youtube.com/watch?v=3tTISzxQ86A

Tchoung Ta Tchen Push hands.m4v , published by Hamish Gordon in the YouTube channel on Dec 10, 2011.

 I have no idea why Hamish Gordon translated 鍾大振 as Tchoung Ta Tchen. In Mandarin 鍾大振 is pronounced as Zhong Dazhen. The above movie shows Mr. Zhong Dazhen's training practice of the Ji form of tai chi power with his push hand partner.

According to the website published by Mr. Zhong's student, Mr. Lee Kam-to 李錦濤 Mr. Zhong 鍾大振 studied qigong in Emei 峨嵋

Mountain, Sichuan 四川 Province, China in 1942. In 1958 he studied Taijiquan with Mr. Shī diào- méi 施調梅 in Taiwan, and practiced push-hand with Mr.鄭曼青 Zheng Manqing. He came to Vancouver in 1972 to set up the Canadian Chinese Tai Chi Association. He was very famous in Vancouver in the 80s and the 90s. He died in 2000 of heart disease in Richmond General Hospital in Vancouver. With the help from Mr. Lee Kam-to Mr. Zhong Dazhen 鍾大振 wrote a tai chi book, 《太極拳體用注解》, which was written in both Chinese and English?

http://www.kamtotaichi.com/Chinese/aboutsifu/ctccac.html

The background post
The
push
hand
training
partner
Mr.
Zhong
Dazhen's
original
position
to start
his ji
form of
power.

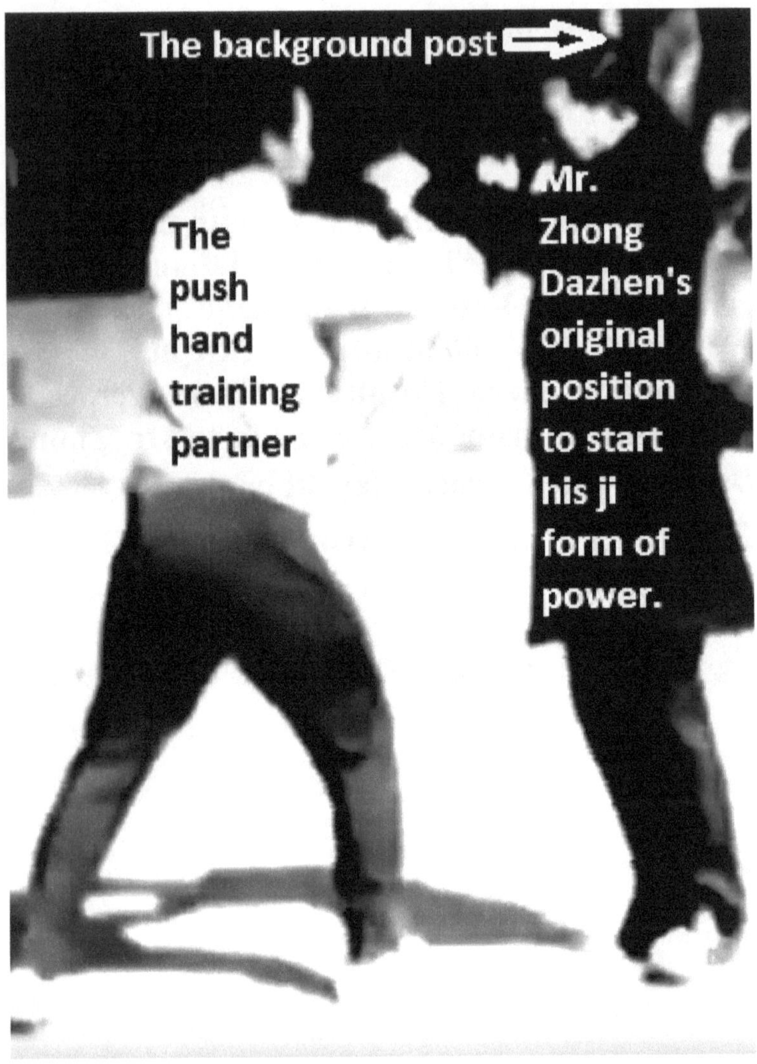

66 dong jin

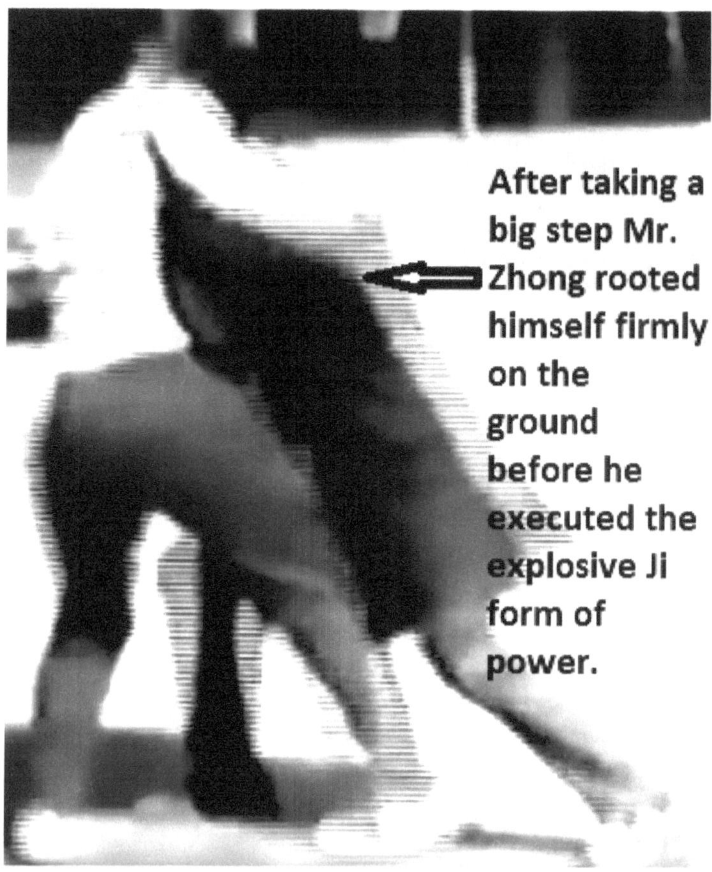

After taking a
big step Mr.
Zhong rooted
himself firmly
on the
ground
before he
executed the
explosive Ji
form of
power.

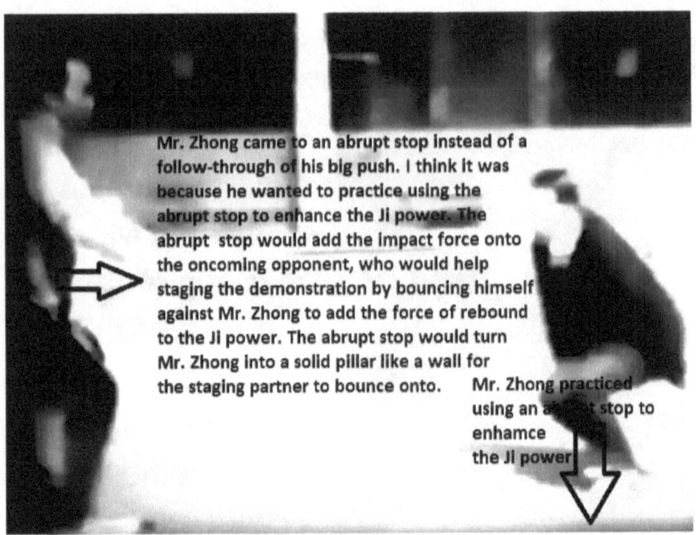

The illustration is magnified below:

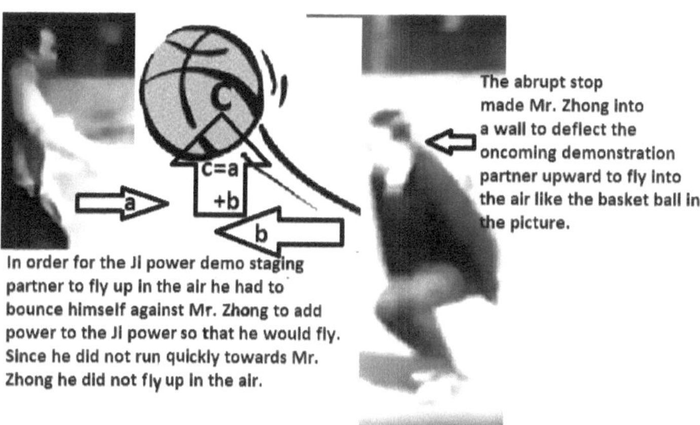

In order for the Ji power demo staging partner to fly up in the air he had to bounce himself against Mr. Zhong to add power to the Ji power so that he would fly. Since he did not run quickly towards Mr. Zhong he did not fly up in the air.

The illustrations are magnified below:

In order for the Ji power demo staging partner to fly up in the air he had to bounce himself against Mr. Zhong to add power to the Ji power so that he would fly. Since he did not run quickly towards Mr. Zhong he did not fly up in the air.

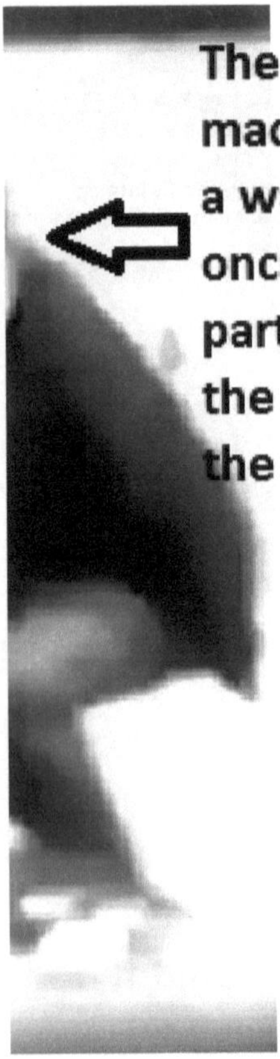

The abrupt stop
made Mr. Zhong into
a wall to deflect the
oncoming demonstration
partner upward to fly into
the air like the basket ball in
the picture.

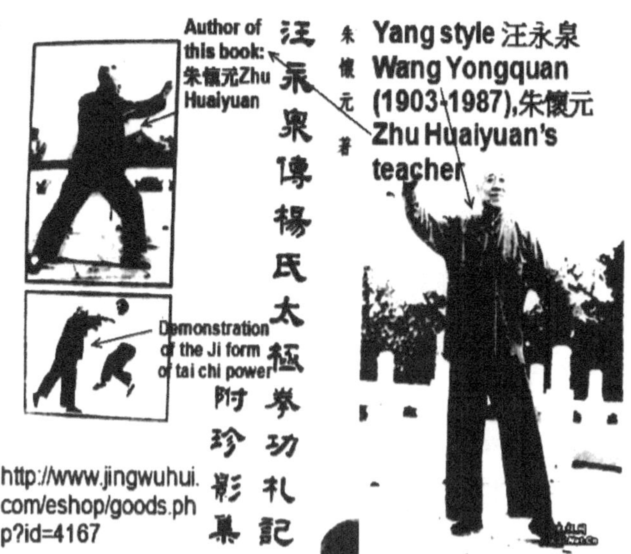

http://www.jingwuhui.
com/eshop/goods.ph
p?id=4167

71 dong jin

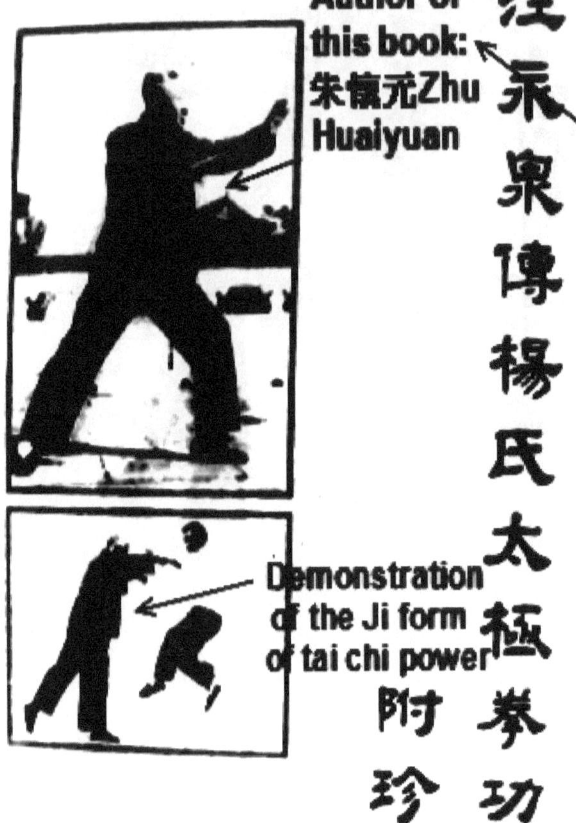

http://www.jingwuhui.com/eshop/goods.p
hp?id=4167

4. The demonstration of the explosive Ji power as shown in the above picture probably originated from the demonstrations by Yang 楊 shǎo hóu 少侯(1862-1930),

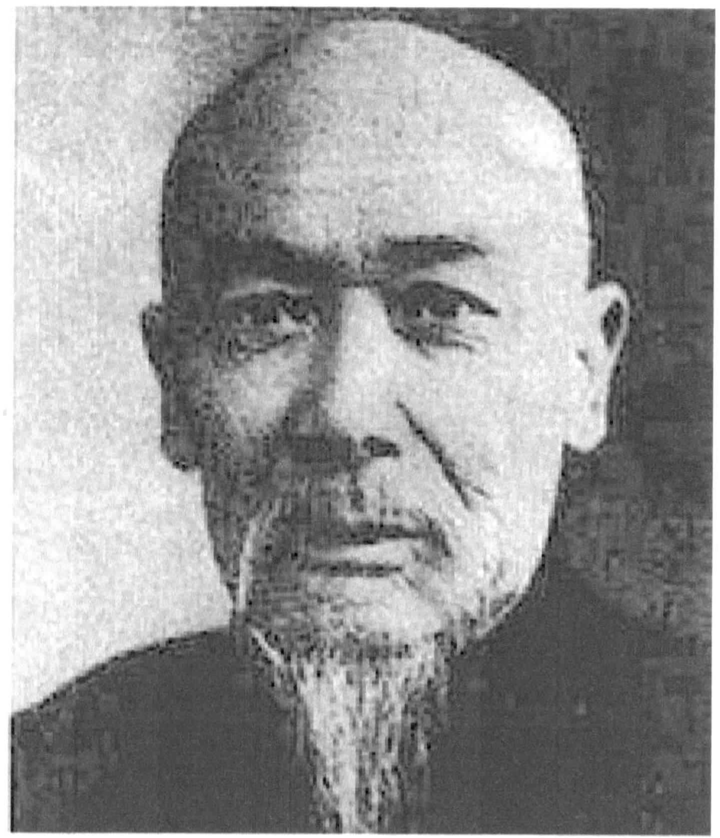

the son of the founder of Yang style tai chi, Yang Lu-chan.

The following two pictures explain the explosive force created in the Ji form of tai chi power:

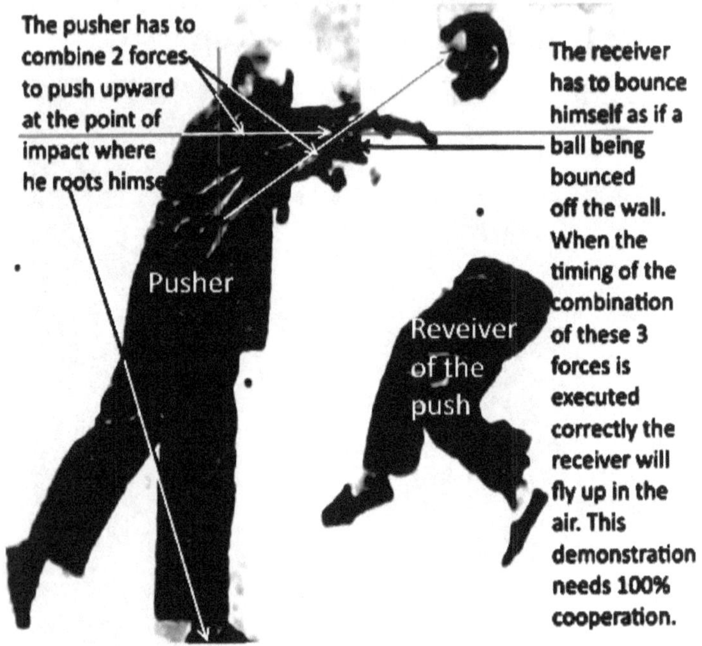

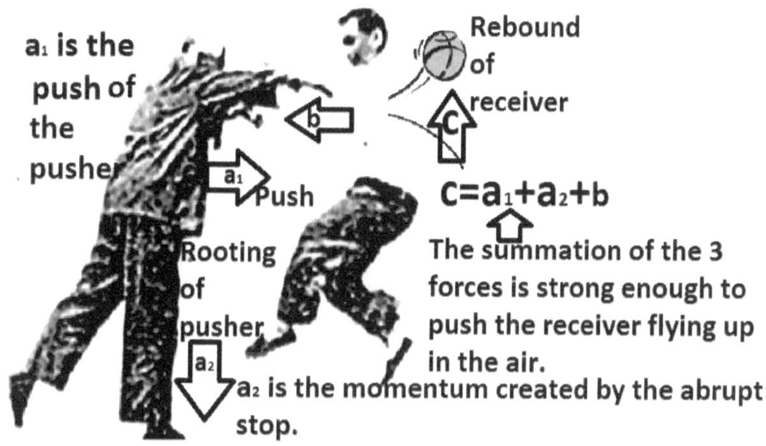

There are quite a lot of similarities between Bruce Lee's explosive one- and six-inch punches and the Ji form of tai chi power. The one inch punch summates the power of the extensions of the elbow, the knee and the momentum created by the sudden abrupt stop of the forward moving body as shown in the above two pictures in the execution of the Ji form of tai chi power. Bruce Lee's power creation also meets the criteria in the "Tai Chi Classics" , "... the power is rooted in the feet; it goes through the legs, controlled by the waist ; it manifested in the fingers. The operation of this power has to be by the body as a whole in all movements. "

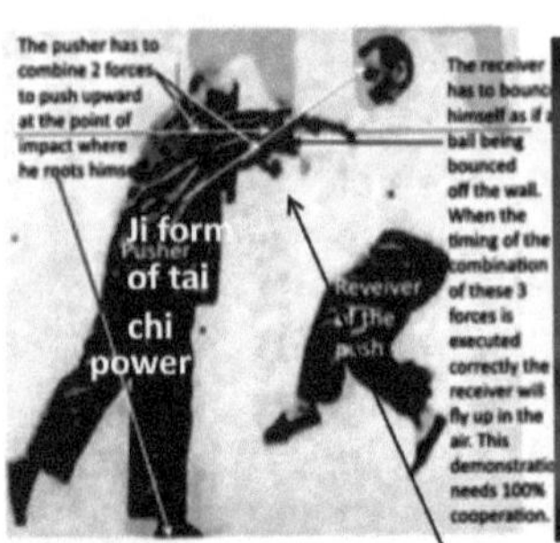

Using the 擠 Ji form of tai chi power to push someone up in the air

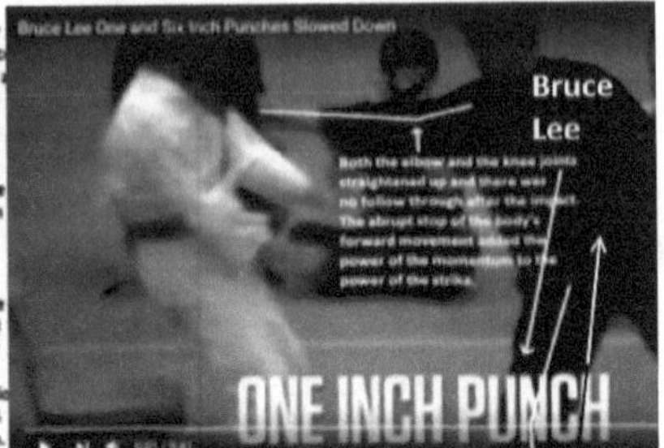

The same principle is used by Bruce Lee in his 1 and 6 inch punches.

The illustration is magnified below:

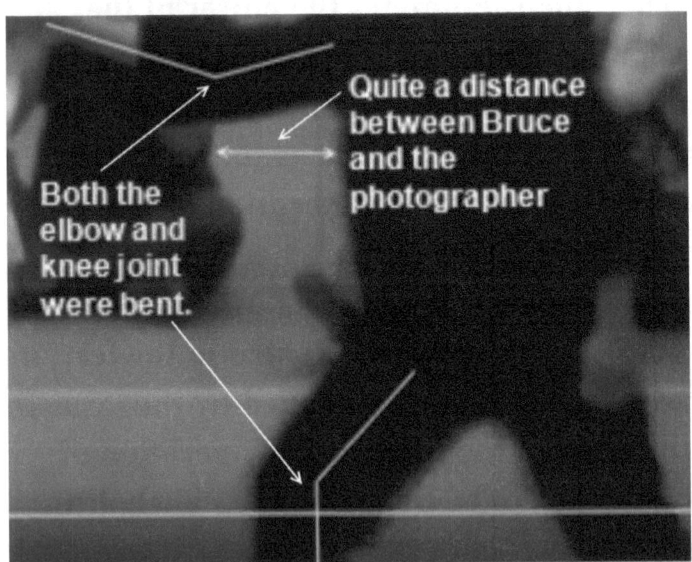

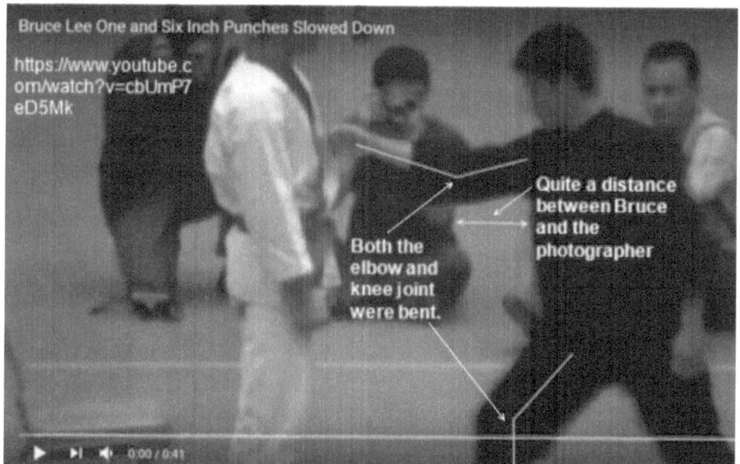

The illustrations are magnified below:

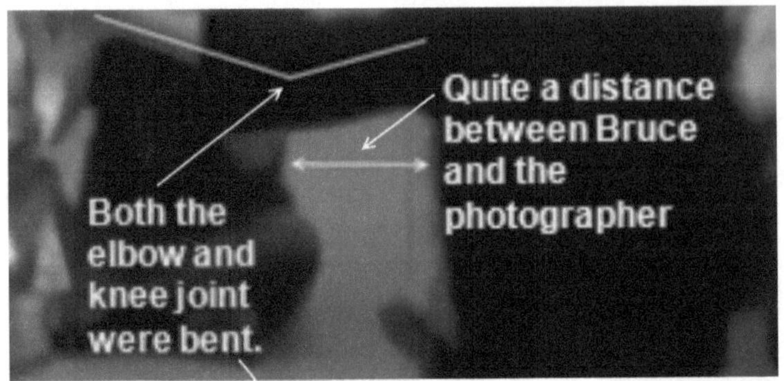

https://www.youtube.com/watch?v=NCfWlYLKJLQBruce lee's one inch punch

https://www.youtube.com/watch?v=

NCfWlYLKJLQBruce lee's one-inch punch

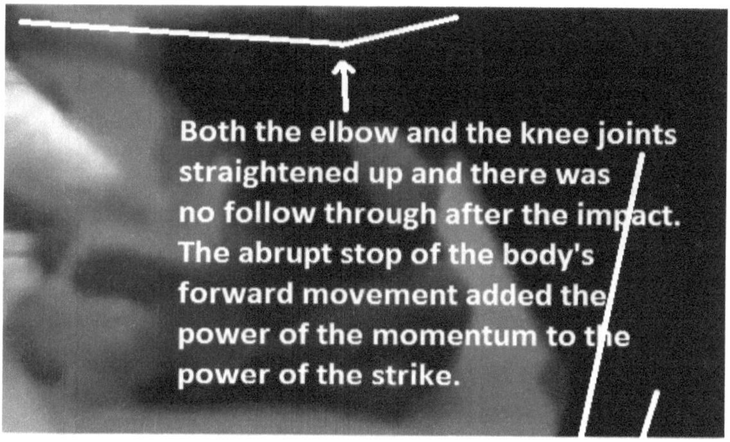

The above illustrations of the enlarged frame of Bruce Lee's one-inch punch shows that it uses the same principle in the Ji form of tai chi power.

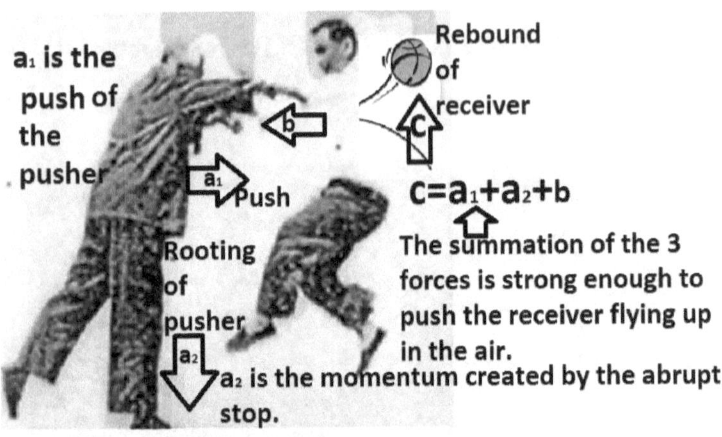

The picture below is taken from a book written by Master 朱懷元 Zhūhuáiyuán《汪永泉傳楊氏太極拳功札記—附珍影集》. Master 朱懷元 Zhūhuáiyuán learned this secret from Master 汪永泉 Wāngyǒngquán .

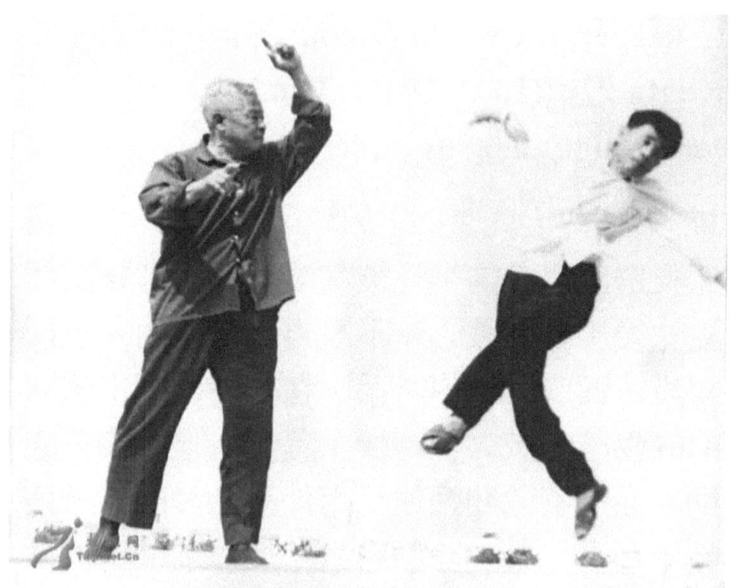

http://www.jingwuhui.com/eshop/goods.php?id=4167

The pusher (Zhu 朱 Huaiyuan 懷元) in the above picture learned this demonstration technique from Wang 汪 Yongquan 永泉 (1903-1987), who seemed to have broken the Chinese tradition and was allowed to learn this martial art secret as an outsider of the Yang style family. He was not related to the Yang style family in anyway and his tai chi training was different from the second generation Yang style

gate-keeper, the world famous Master Yang 楊 Chengfu 澄甫(1883–1936). The following records might help us understand:

當時，人稱"大先生"的少侯公出手不留情，發勁兇狠是出了名的。凡被其淩空拋出者嘗到個中滋味後，都膽戰心驚不敢再靠前。而永泉則經常設法與少侯師伯試手，在被發挨摔中體驗師伯的勁路、威力與時機、奧妙。但始終只能聽勁，從來不敢問師伯是用什麼勁發的。一連十數年耳濡目染，身領心悟。加之前期有健侯公指點，後期有嚴父教誨，故永泉公深得楊家內功勁法之真傳，尤其在揉手方面很有造詣。在後來的幾十年?，他始終堅持早年和父親一道從健侯公所學的老六路拳架的原始練法，所習、所傳拳架與楊師澄甫南下上海等地所教的套路動作及練法不一。

http://taijiwenwutang.blogspot.ca/2006/02/blog-post_09.html

The following is my translation of the above except:

Yang 楊 shǎo hóu 少侯, also called bān hóu 班侯 was one of the two sons of the founder of Yang style tai chi, Yang 楊 Lù chán 露禪（1799－1872）. He was making a living teaching tai chi to some of the imperial members of the Qing Dynasty. In order to demonstrate the power of his kung fu his training partners were often thrown hard and because of frequent injuries that happened during his demonstrations nobody dared to act as the demonstration partner except Wang 汪 Yongquan 永泉, who was very good at Manchurian wrestling and knew how to fall without sustaining too many injuries. In many tai chi demonstrations like the aforementioned Ji power, a 100% total cooperation from the partner was a must. This was why Wang 汪 Yongquan 永泉 was able to learn the Yang style kung fu family secret as a demonstration partner of Yang 楊 shǎo hóu 少侯, who had no choice because his only immediate family member, his nephew, Yang 楊 Chengfu 澄甫 did not want to learn tai chi the hard way, to be thrown around in those demonstrations and be injured frequently.

There is why Wang 汪 Yongquan 永泉's style of the Yang tai chi is called the "Lǎo liùlù" 老六路, which literally means the "old six roads". It is different from Yang 楊 Chengfu 澄甫's style of tai chi in spite of the fact that Wang 汪 Yongquan also studied from Yang 楊 Chengfu 澄甫, who learned his tai chi after his grandfather, Yang 楊 Lù chán 露禪 died. His uncle bān hóu 班侯（1837 年－1892 年）、and his father jiànhóu 楊健侯 were very old. His tai chi was literally self taught and was called the "large frame" or "Da Jia (大架)" with expansive footwork coupling with smooth and large circular hand and arm motions. It was probably because of this self-learning experience Master Yang Chengfu 楊澄甫 (1883－1936) wrote a very popular book , called "Tài Jí quán tǐ yòng quán shū 太極拳體

用全書" in 1934.

"鬆開 Song kai" was one of the key principles in Tai Chi that was heavily emphasized by Master Chengfu Yang

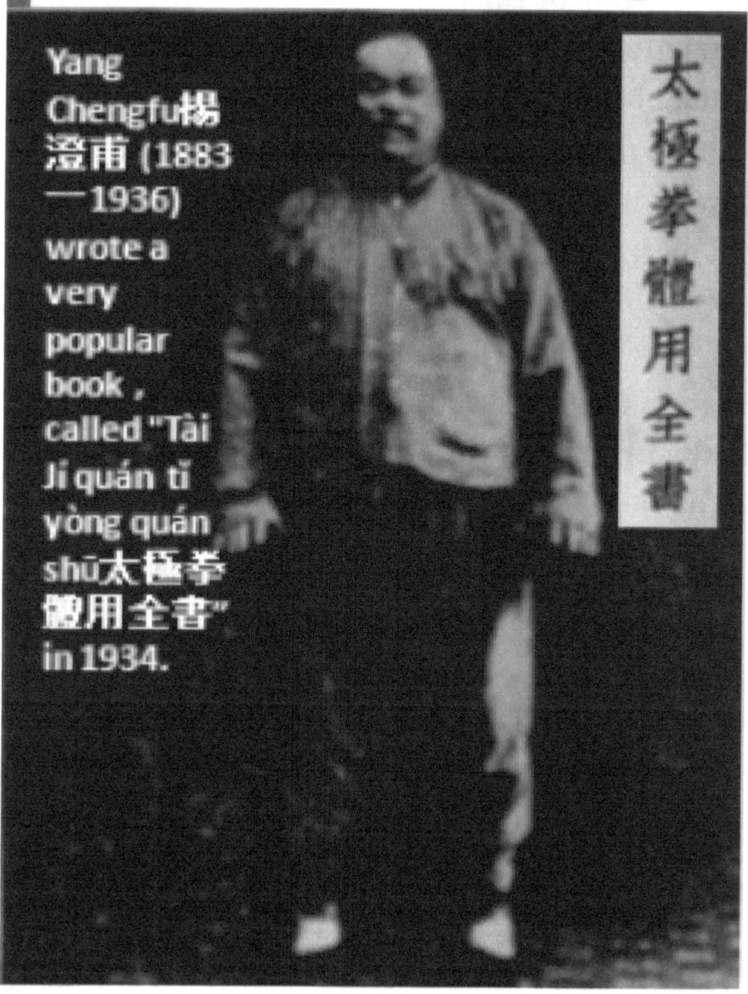

"Tǐ 體" means the invisible internal essence and "yòng 用" means the externally visible expressions of the functions. According to Yang Chengfu's world famous student, Master Cheng Manqing (Cheng 鄭 Manqing 曼青 1902 - 1975) there had been at least one recorded case of a man who had successfully learned tai chi on his own with this book.

Master Cheng Manqing wrote about this case in the preface of his book, Zhèng zi tàijí quán zìxiū xīnfǎ 鄭子太極拳自修新法.

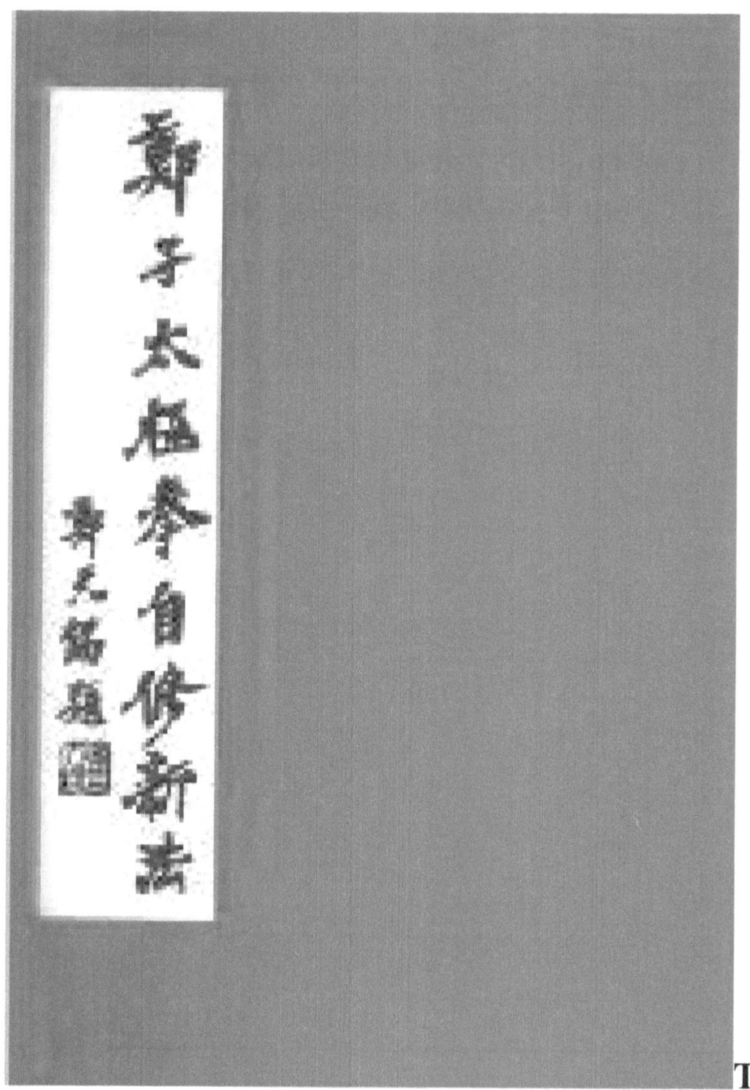

his book was translated into English by Mr. Louis Swaim and published by North Atlantic

Books in 2005. The title in English is, , "The Essence and Applications of Taijiquan".

You can compare the two versions of the Yang style tai chi yourself to see the difference.

https://www.youtube.com/watch?v=YBrwGG9gSPs

Yang Family Taijiquan - Master Wang Yongquan

5.To have the privilege of inheriting the Yang style kung fu secret Wang 汪 Yongquan 永泉 (1904-1987) paid dearly when you see how he suffered in his old age.

https://www.youtube.com/watch?v=hz7AGjWcDxs

Wang Yongquan Full Fajing Demo

At 4.44 of the above movie you can see him sitting on a chair and was still able to use his tai chi Ji power to push people off the ground a little bit.

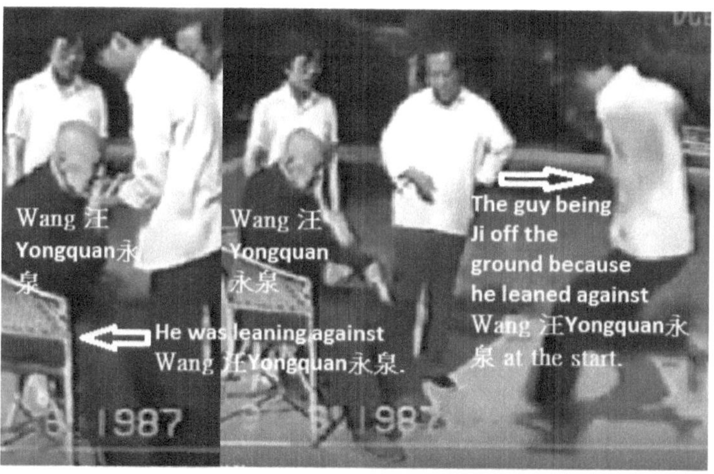

The illustrations are magnified below:

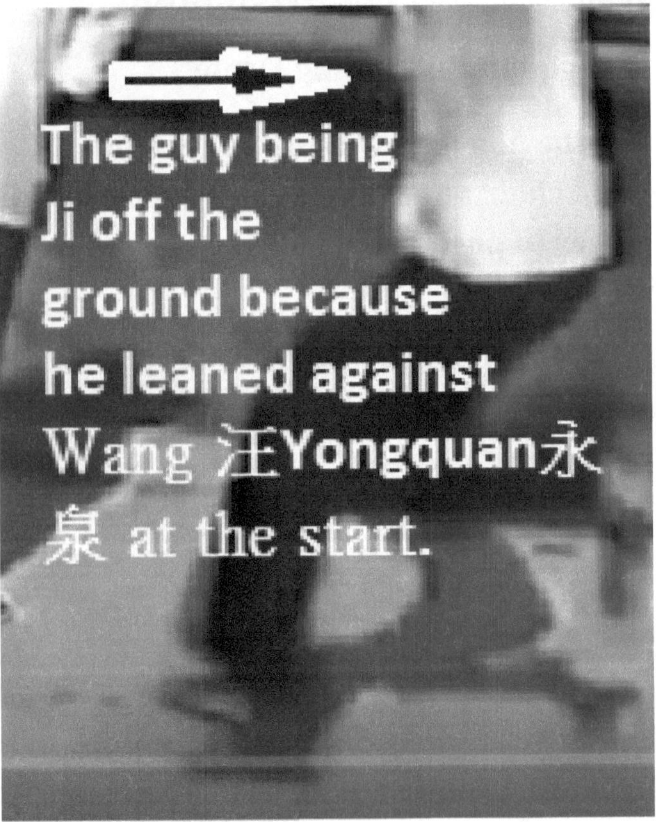
He was leaning against
Wang 汪 Yongquan 永泉.
The guy being
Ji off the
ground because
he leaned against
Wang 汪 Yongquan 永
泉 at the start.

But at 0.47- 0.53 of the same movie you can see him being helped bilaterally to stand upright in spite of the fact that he was carrying a cane. I do not think he could walk on his own.

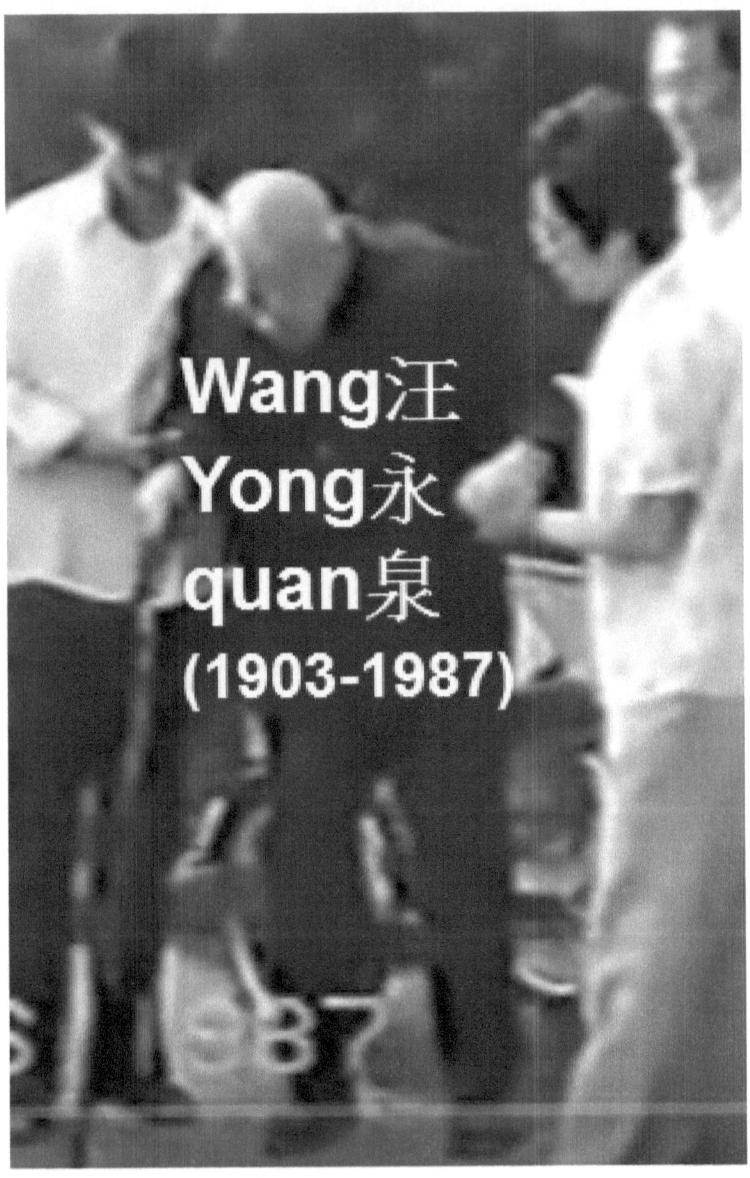

92 dong jin

The possible cause of Wang 汪 Yongquan 永泉's disability:

Repeated small injuries to the low back during practice can cause some severe spinal injuries. Initially some hairline bone fractures appear with very minor pain symptoms of local pain, which subsides with rest. When ignored the hairline bone fracture will become a real bone fracture. When a bone fracture occurs at the narrow bone connection, called the pars interarticalaris that joins the vertebral arch and the vertebral body the whole spinal column will slide forward, compressing the spinal nerve and cause leg pain and walking difficulty as seen in the case of Wang 汪 Yongquan 永泉.

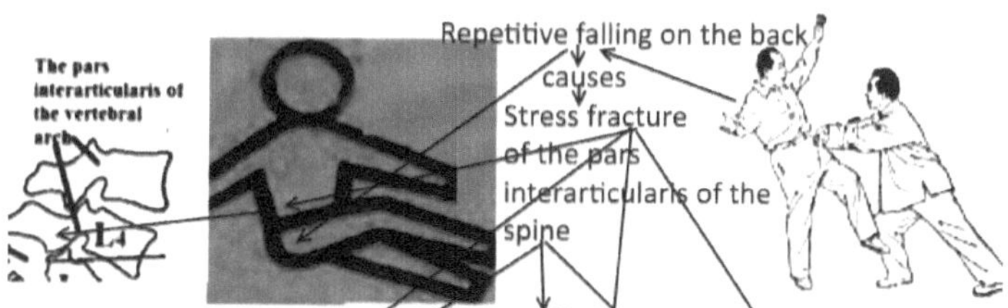

The illustrations are magnified below:

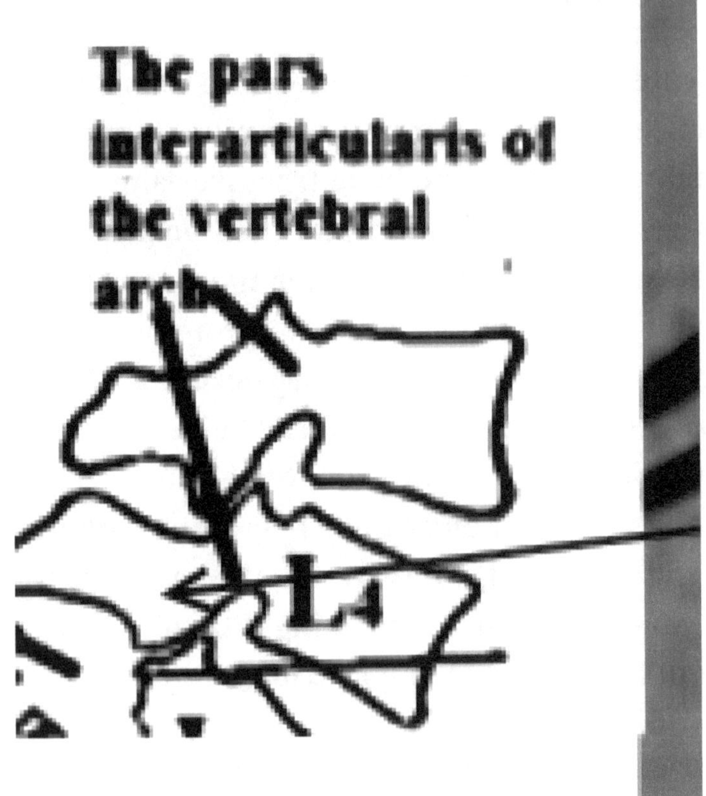
The pars
interarticularis of
the vertebral
arch
L4

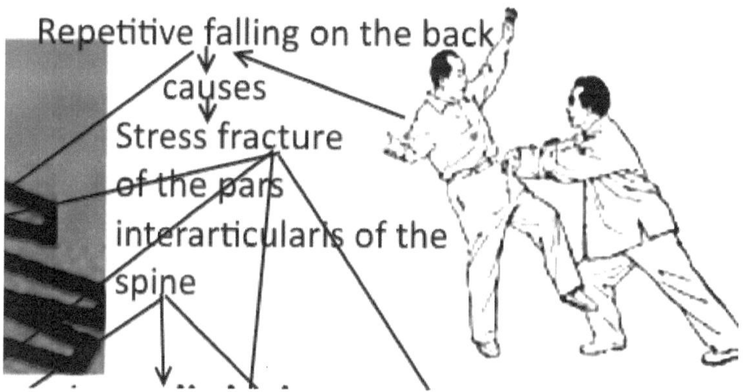

Stress fractures, also known as hairline fractures, are fatigue-induced fractures of the bone caused by repeated stress over time. Instead of resulting from a single severe impact, stress fractures are the result of accumulated trauma from repeated submaximal loading, such as running or jumping. Because of this mechanism, stress fractures are common overuse injuries in athletes. [1. Behrens, Steve; Deren, Matson; Fadale, Monchik (March–April 2013). "Stress Fractures of the Pelvis and Legs in Athletes". Sports Health: A Multidisciplinary Approach. 5 (2): 165–174.

doi:10.1177/1941738112467423. Retrieved 2014-05-19.]

Stress fractures can be described as a very small sliver or crack in the bone;[2."Stress fractures - MayoClinic.com". Retrieved 2007-12-23.] and are sometimes referred to as "hairline fractures". https://en.wikipedia.org/wiki/Stress_fracture

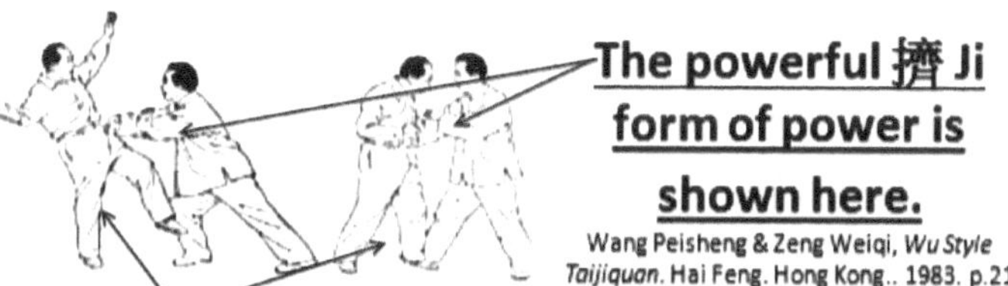

Wang Peisheng & Zeng Weiqi, *Wu Style Taijiquan*. Hai Feng. Hong Kong.. 1983. p.21

- **The receiver has to cooperate by sustaining the power 100% and this is why the risk of injuries is high during practices, especially among enthusiastic but not quite accomplished tai chi practitioners. Shoulder injuries and rib fracture can happen easily.**

- **Serious spinal injuries like anterolisthesis can occur too.**

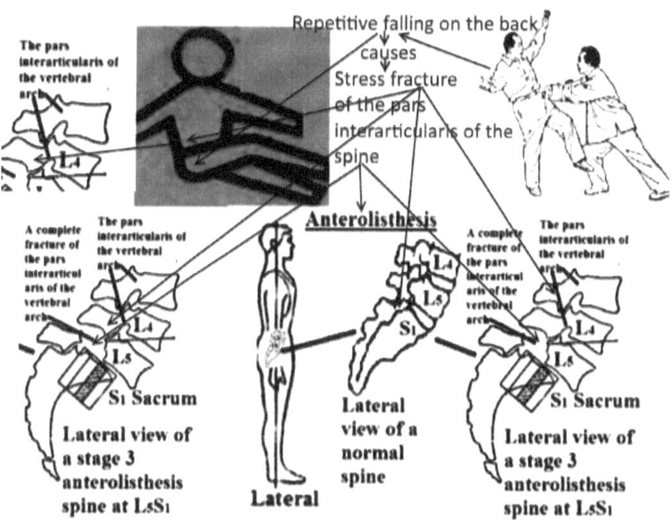

The illustrations are magnified below:

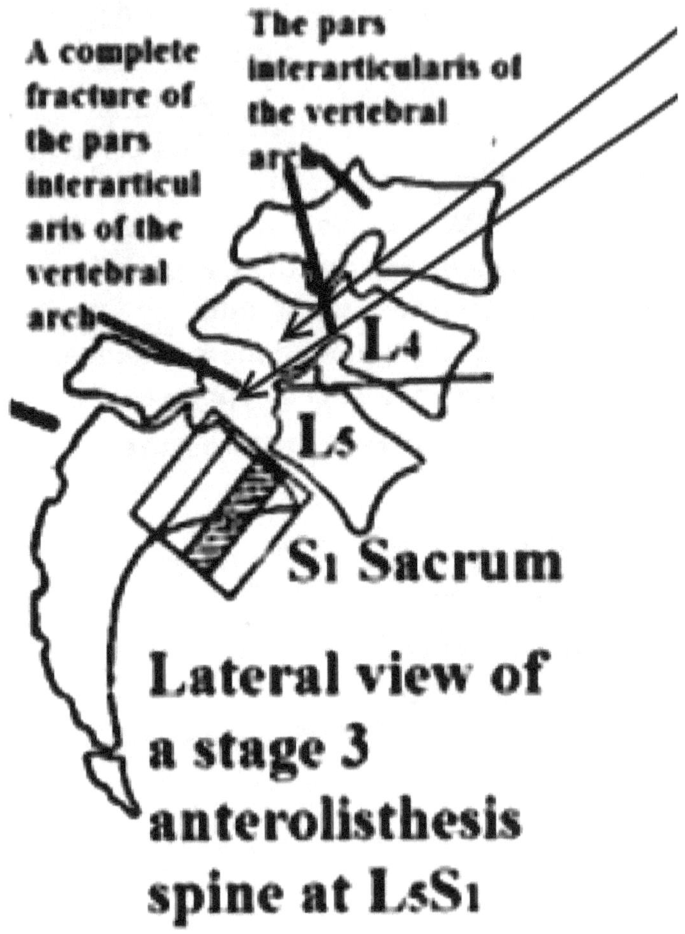

A complete fracture of the pars interarticul aris of the vertebral arch
The pars interarticularis of the vertebral arch
L4
L5
S1 Sacrum
Lateral view of a stage 3 anterolisthesis spine at L5S1

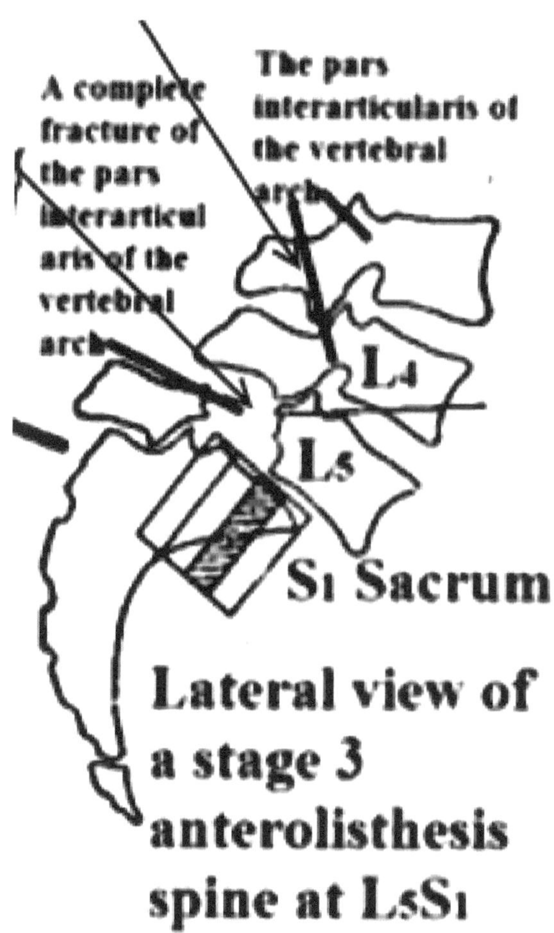

A complete fracture of the pars interarticularis of the vertebral arch
The pars interarticularis of the vertebral arch
L4
L5
S1 Sacrum
Lateral view of a stage 3 anterolisthesis spine at L5S1

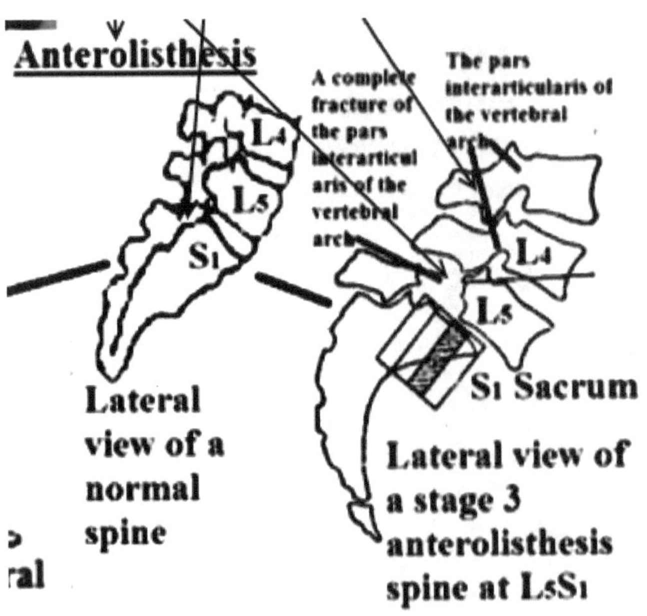

Anterolisthesis
L4
L5
S1
Lateral view of a normal spine
A complete fracture of the pars interarticularis of the vertebral arch
The pars interarticularis of the vertebral arch
L4
L5
S1 Sacrum
Lateral view of a stage 3 anterolisthesis spine at L5S1

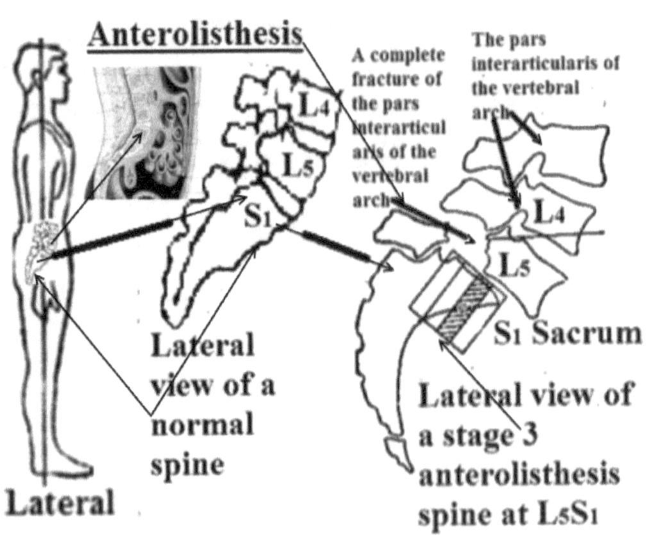

Anterolisthesis
L4
L5
S1
Lateral
Lateral view of a normal spine
A complete fracture of the pars interarticularis of the vertebral arch
The pars interarticularis of the vertebral arch
L4
L5
S1 Sacrum
Lateral view of a stage 3 anterolisthesis spine at L5S1

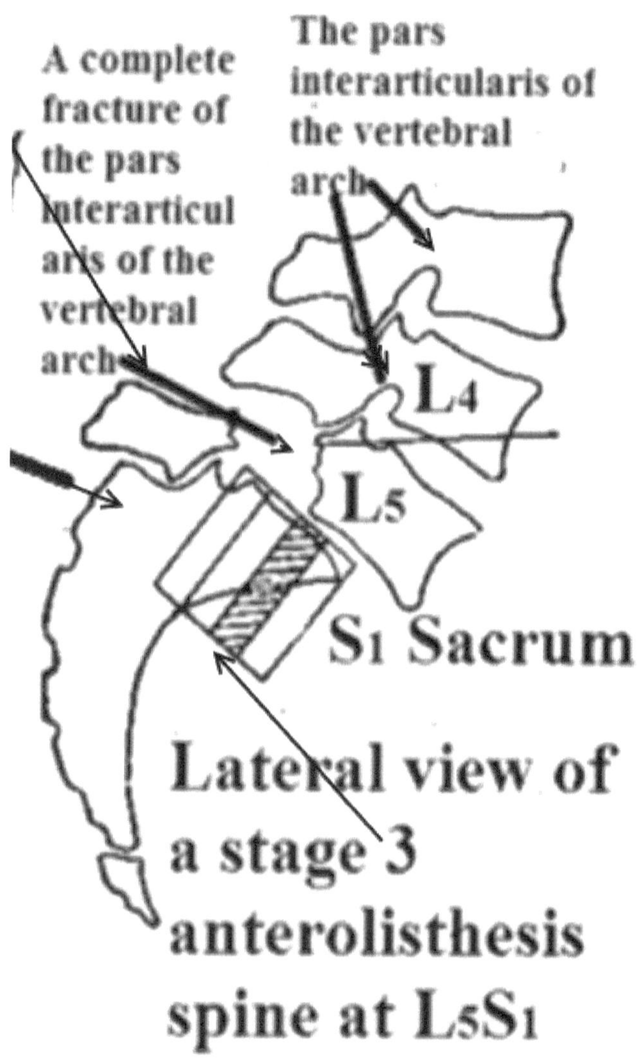

The illustration is magnified below:

101 dong jin

Signs and symptoms of anterolisthesis include

1/ Weakness of the legs and this may or may not be accompanied by numbness.

2/ Tingling

3/ Inability to control the legs

4/Abnormal sensations

5/. Inability to control the passage of urine or bowel movements

Wang 汪 Yongquan 永泉's disability presentation in the above movie shows the sign of weakness of the legs bilaterally. With his history of repetitive heavy and abusive usage of the low back in pushing and resisting pushes and punches my speculation of his disability might be right.

In my three decades of chiropractic practice I have found a way to reduce anterolisthesis non-surgically and noninvasively, using tai chi power in the application of external spinal manipulation. However, I would like to have this technique verified academically and then I can teach it to qualified professionals to be executed under safe and insured circumstances.

6.I have one more negative feeling of this dangerous and rather fake way to demonstrate the Ji form of power. I witnessed this unethical use of the Ji form of power personally by a tai chi teacher, who used this Ji form of power in a very unethical manner to advertise his kung fu. I was in one of the public parks of Vancouver, called the Queen Elizabeth Park. There was one group of people learning tai chi from a tai chi teacher. The aforementioned tai chi teacher mysteriously appeared and went towards that tai chi teacher asking for a friendly round of push hand. Then without any warning he suddenly used the Ji form of power the same way as shown in the above movie to push the tai chi teacher on the ground. After embarrassing the tai chi teacher in front of his student and in a public area he had the nerve to hypocritically apologize to that teacher, who was being insulted right in front of his students. However, people witnessing this were impressed with that tai chi teacher's tai chi power. That was one of his ways to publicize himself.

In old China, kung fu masters were often challenged by new instructors and a certain disclaimer was usually signed before a kung fu contest. It is regarded as unethical to stage a challenge without any warning. If an unprovoked attack was staged to hurt another established martial artist to gain fame the challenger would be scorned at and looked down upon. However, in the Western world that does not have this ancient Chinese tradition kung fu and tai chi instructors might be able to use this kind of unethical methods and get away with it.

Mr. Zhong Dazhen 鍾大振 became well-known as a tai chi master with "real" push hand kung fu in Vancouver and he made a good living teaching tai chi until he died. Is he a good teacher? Please use your judgement.

Mr. Zhong Dazhen 鍾大振 had another way to impress people. Once in a while he would demonstrate his ability to resist the push of a linear and long line of people as shown in the picture below. He did that in the 80s and the 90s and many people were very impressed. Even nowadays there are tai chi masters using this trick technique to impress people who do not know tai chi that well. Many were and are very impressed with this trick technique. But people who know tai chi well would scorn at this trick technique because the main idea of tai chi is to go with the flow of any incoming force, which is absolved or redirected back to the opponent. If you look at the picture below you will realize that it is a trick demonstration.

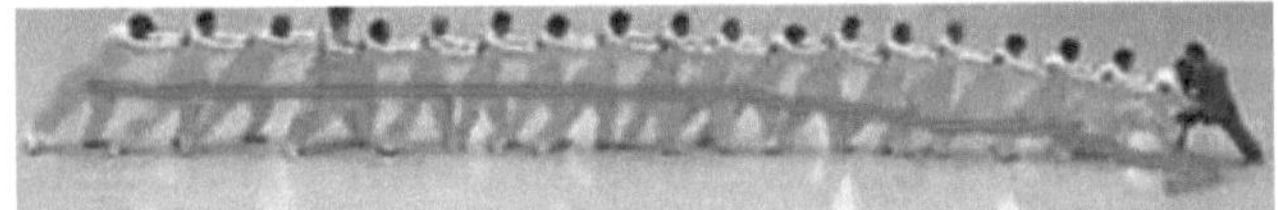

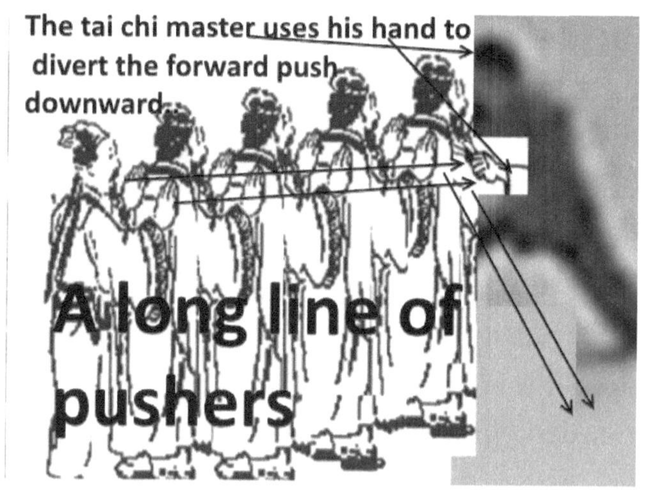

The tai chi master demonstrating this trick uses the first person of that long line of people to re-direct all the power downward. Please view this movie in terms of the aforementioned explanations to see for yourself:

https://www.youtube.com/watch?v=O0Z3Zhj8ICY

太极拳之"千斤坠"，不知道外国人看到这个会相信么？

It is that first person absolving most of the power. The line of people can be very long

but it is hard to synchronize their pushing together so that all the power is used in that push. This linear long line of people is already a obvious sign that it is a trick demonstration set up. It is impressive but it is definitely not real kung fu and definitely not tai chi kung fu because in tai chi if one resist a push it is called double weight. In Chinese it is called 雙重則滯, which means that it will become stagnation when both forces are going head to head against each other. (王宗岳 Wángzōngyuè was a legendary figure in the history of t'ai chi ch'uan (taijiquan). In some writings, Wang was a famous student of the legendary Zhang Sanfeng, a 13th-century Taoist monk credited with devising neijia in general and t'ai chi ch'uan in particular.

https://en.wikipedia.org/wiki/Wang_Zongyue:...偏沉則隨，雙重則滯。每見數年純功，不能運化者，率皆自為人制，雙重之病未悟耳。欲避此病，須知陰陽。黏即是走，走即是黏。陰不離陽，陽不離陰，陰陽相濟，方

為懂勁。懂勁後愈練愈精，默識揣摩，漸至
從心所欲。）

My translation of the above tai chi classics:

When you resist the oncoming force, you stagnate the mutually complementary yin-yang principle of change in tai chi. When the ongoing yin-yang principle of change is stopped it is called Shuāngchóng 雙重, which literally means double weight in Chinese. Instead of resisting the oncoming force neutralize it by directing and following it sideway or downward with your newly acquired tai chi adhesive reflex, which has the built-in yin-yang principle of change. If you can manipulate tai chi power with this adhesive yin-yang principle of change you have reached a superior stage of kung fu sophistication. In Chinese it is called Dǒng jìn 懂勁, which literally means understanding the power. Once you have reached Dǒng jìn 懂勁 you can teach and improve your kung fu on your own by experimenting this new reflex of movements and gradually this

new movement-reflex becomes natural and operates without your conscious thinking.

Seeing Mr. Zhong's demonstration of double weight and his sudden attack on the push-hand opponent in a so-called friendly game of push-hand I have a lot of doubt of the ethical value of Mr. Zhong as a martial art teacher.

7.There are ways to discredit the above two unethical ways to use tai chi power to advertise one's tai chi kung fu.

When anyone who wants to deliver a sudden push with the Ji power, he has to take a big step towards you as shown in the following picture. Then you can get ready to use the Cai or the Lu form of power to teach him a lesson. With the Cai form of power, he will be thrown to the ground right in front of you and with the Lu form of power he will be swung to the side. If you have a strong rooting stance you do not even have to take a step backward to execute these two forms of power. Any tai chi master with real tai chi kung fu can demonstrate these techniques, which are useful when you do push hand with people you do not know too well. Just get ready if he takes a step towards you.

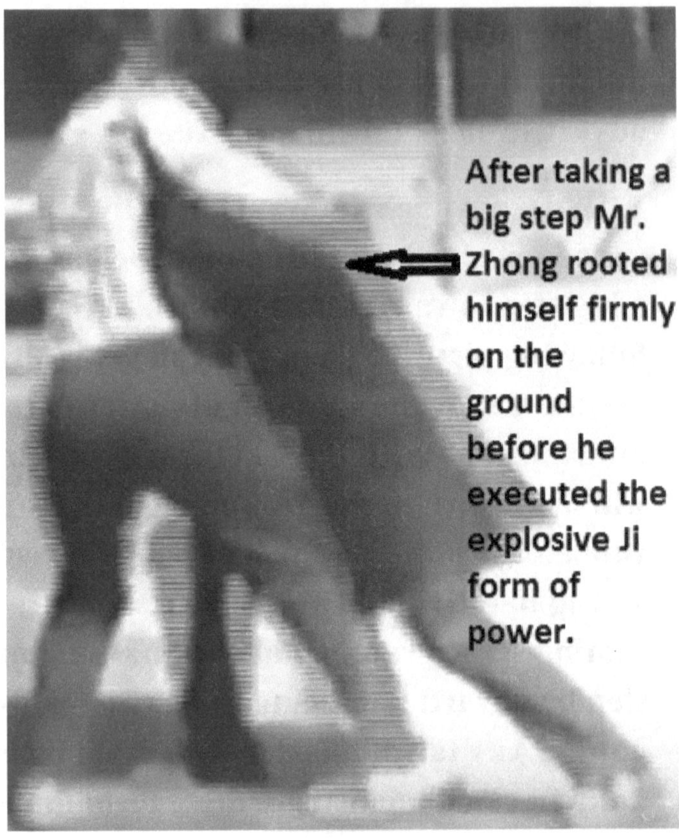

The Ji form of power can be defeated by the Cai or the An form of power as shown:

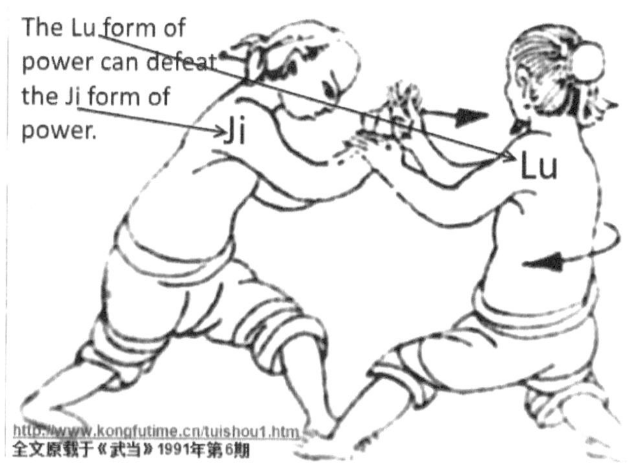

The Lu form of power can defeat the Ji form of power.
Ji
Lu
http://www.kongfutime.cn/tuishou1.htm
全文原载于《武当》1991年第6期

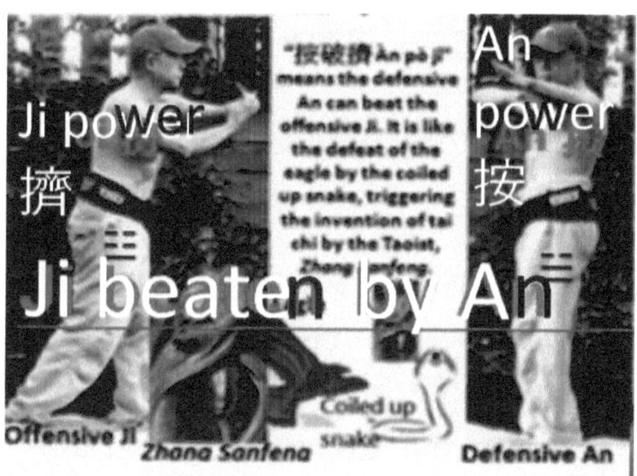

Ji power
擠
Ji beaten by An
Offensive Ji
Zhana Sanfena
"按破擠 àn pò jǐ" means the defensive An can beat the offensive Ji. It is like the defeat of the eagle by the coiled up snake, triggering the invention of tai chi by the Taoist, Zhang Sanfeng.
An power
按
Coiled up snake
Defensive An

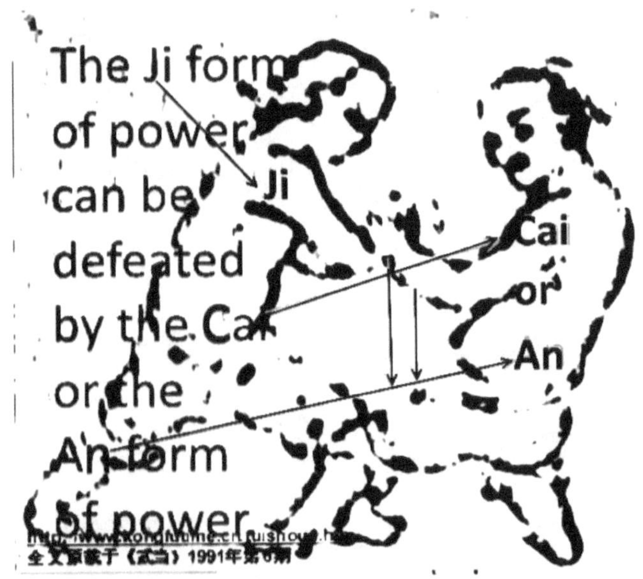

To demystify the long line of people pushing trick:

Instead of pushing the so-called master with two hands supported by the power of a long line of people just ask to push him with two to three people facing him with four to six hands on his body and I think a fake tai chi demonstrator depending on his performance with the above trick technique will probably cancel the demonstration because he knows that he cannot manipulate all the four or six hands with only his two

hands to direct all the four to six forces downward to the ground.

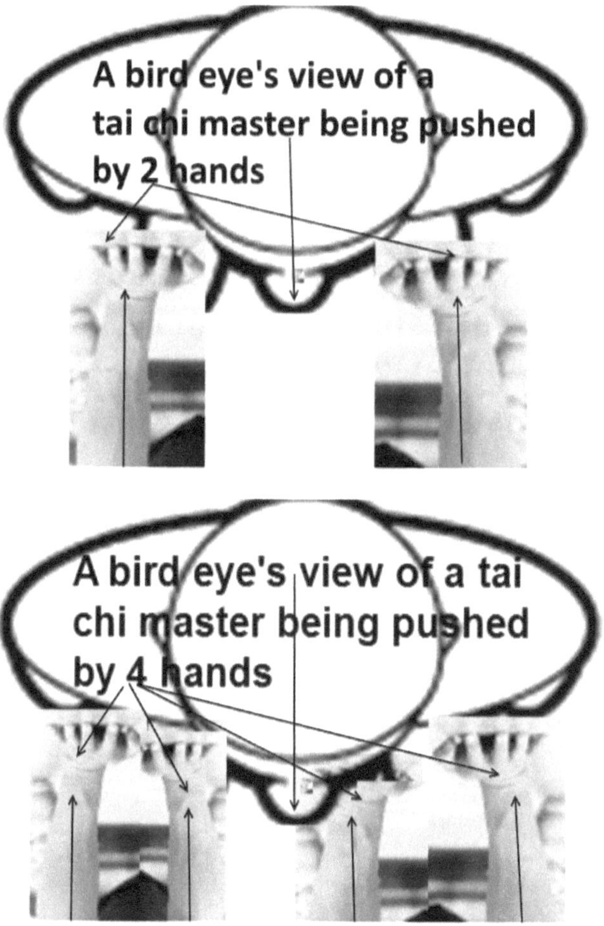

The above two techniques have been used for several decades to demonstrate tai chi power.

However, in this internet age it is impossible to fool all the people all the time.

I have another observation. None of Zhong Dazhen's students has demonstrated the two aforementioned tai chi exhibition "skills" of throwing people up in the air and resisting the push of a long line of people. Perhaps these techniques are very difficult to understand and to practice. His students cannot master them. However, I think Zhong Dazhen took the secrets with him to the grave because he knew these methods were just tricks. If his students knew these secrets they would not respect him.

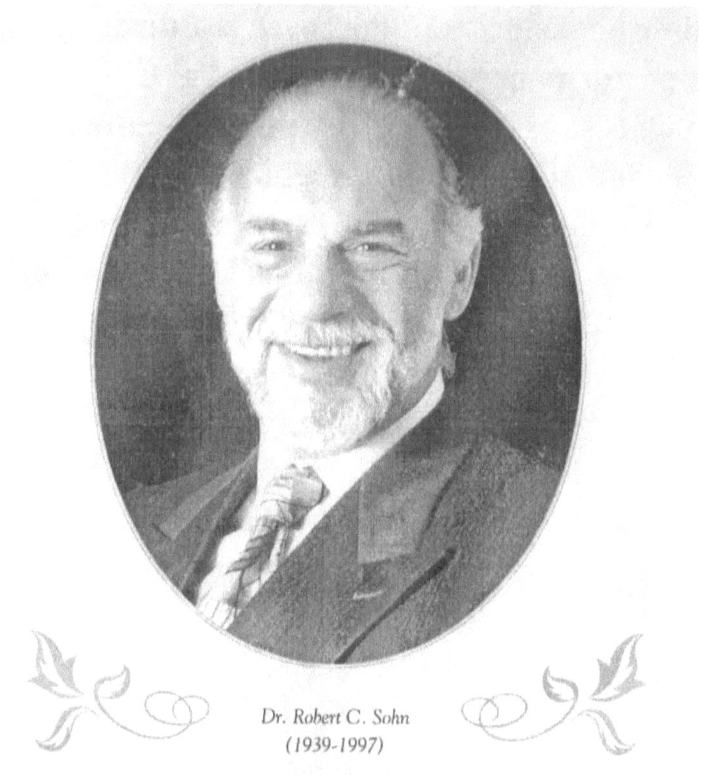

Dr. Robert C. Sohn
(1939-1997)

Http://www.w1ndhorse.com/agreatman.html

Contemporary with Zhong Dazhen a Westerner tai chi practitioner, Dr. Robert C. Sohn (acupuncturist, 1939, - 1997 as shown in the picture) wrote a tai chi kung fu book titled Tao and T'ai Chi Kung, published in 1987, by Destiny Books. It is available in the Amazon

online bookstore. On the cover is a drawing of his performance the immovable Tai Chi stance, which is substantiated by a photo-picture in p.36, and another photo-picture, described as the unliftable stance in p.38). Dr. Robert C. Sohn died in 1997 at the young age of 58 and the cause of death has not been reported. There is not a single report of a successor of his T'ai Chi Kung, which according to him is a combination of martial art and Taoist yoga, a combination of his own creation. In the book, he reveals a series of exercises to train practitioners to straighten the spine (p.107-112 in the book). On p.112 there is a lateral display of his cervical (neck) X-ray picture to show that he has practiced his T'ai Chi Kung to the sophisticated level to have acquired a straight cervical spine. In some of my YouTube movies and my self-published essays I have repeatedly advised tai chi and qigong practitioners not to practise any techniques to flatten the three spinal curves because they have important functions. Shock absorption is an obvious one. In a nutshell, is Robert C. Sohn's immovable stance good for health? Doubtful! Is there any practical value? The answer is no.

After my scientific explanations of the formation of the Ji form of tai chi power readers should know that it is inadequate to translate Ji as Squeeze or Squeeze forward. It is a sudden push enhanced by the momentum, created by a sudden stop of the pusher. If you call this squeezing or squeezing energy it will lead to many misinterpretations.

8. **The above principle of combining the forward momentum of the pusher with the pushing force was probably originally conceived of by Master 郭 Guō 雲深 yúnshēn (1829－1900) of 形意 xíng yì when he was imprisoned for three years, during when his feet were shackled and hands were handcuffed as shown:**

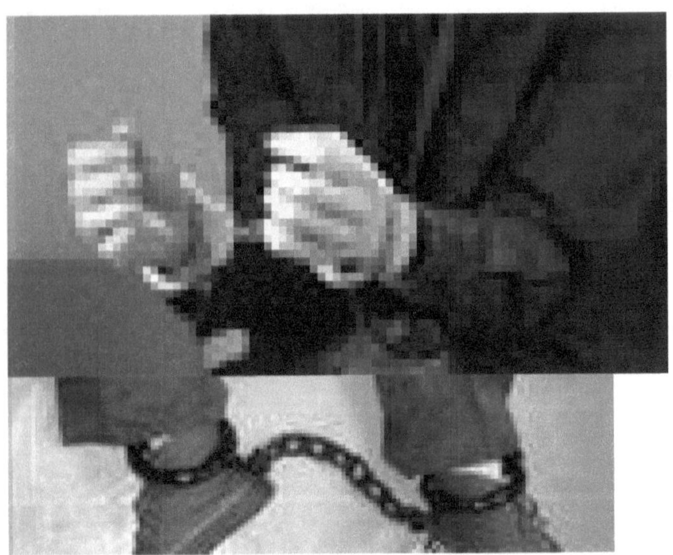

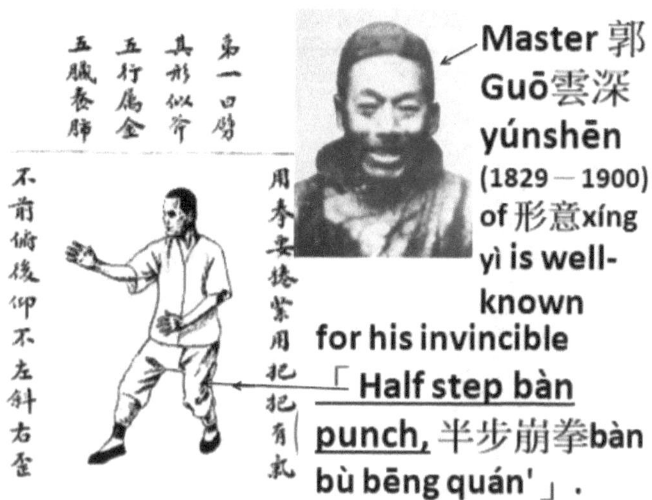

Master Guo's famous invincible "Half step ban punch is demonstrated by his famous student, Master Sun Lutong:

Half step bēng punch, in Chinese 半步崩拳 **bàn bù bēng quán**

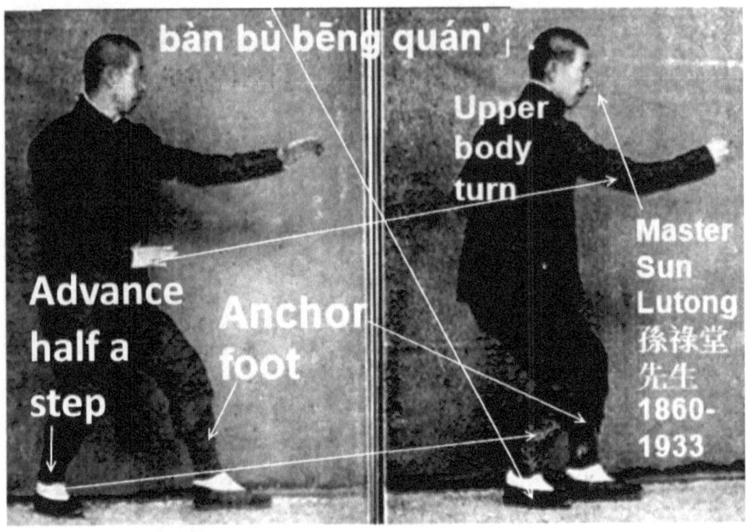

Instead of using his martial arts power in his kung fu demonstration Master Guo was a well-known good fighter and was known to be able to knock out his opponents in one punch.

Master Sun is even more famous than Master Guo as a fighter as well as an Enlightened Daoist practitioner. Details of his Enlightenment is in my Kindle ebook,

> "The path to Enlightenment from the practice of Tai Chi + 站椿 Zhàn zhuāng (pile stance): The Shen Ming of Tai Ch is

the complementary component of your meditation for Enlightenment"

https://www.amazon.com/dp/B07DZNVWZ5

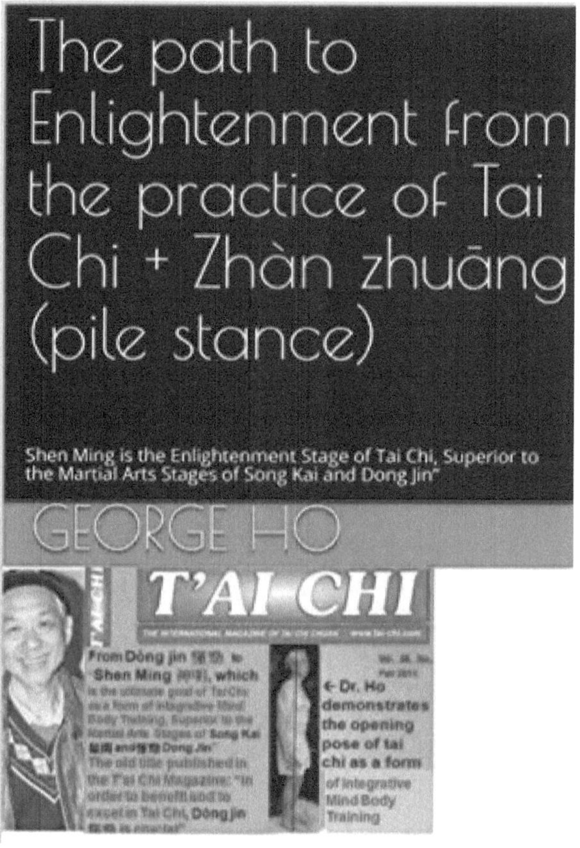

123 dong jin

9. The following ways of using the tennis serve and the tennis strokes are some of my suggestions to train and to evaluate one's tai chi power in fa jin, 發勁, which means firing the power of tai chi.

In the following picture I have compared a tennis serve to the punch used by Wu Gong-yi, the second-generation gatekeeper of Wu style tai chi in an arena fight.

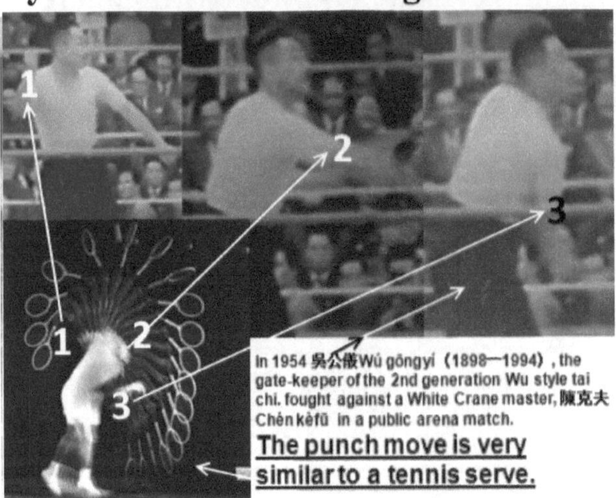

In 1954 吳公儀 Wú gōngyí (1898—1994) , the gate-keeper of the 2nd generation Wu style tai chi. fought against a White Crane master, 陳克夫 Chén kèfū in a public arena match. The punch move is very similar to a tennis serve.

The illustration is magnified below:

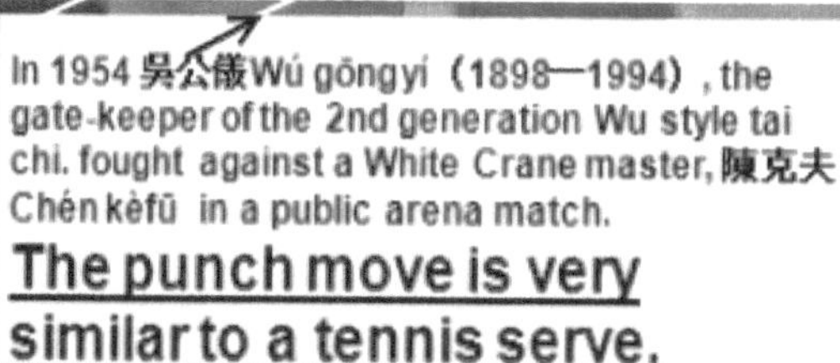

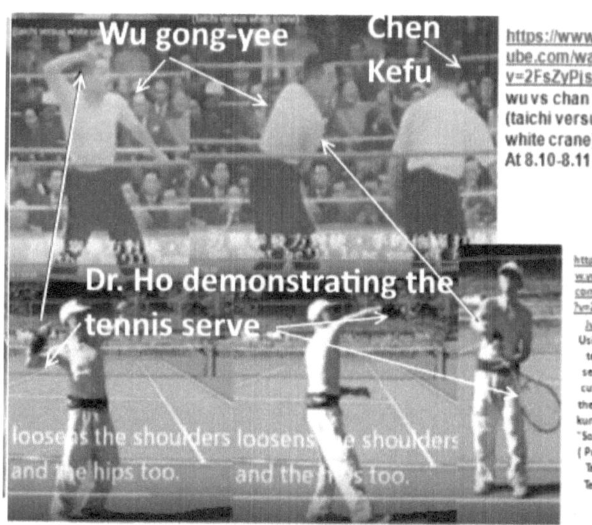

The fight between him and a White Crane martial artist was in Macau in 1954. The movie of the fight has been uploaded onto YouTube; the link is
https://www.youtube.com/watch?v=2FsZyPjsjTA

wu vs chan 1954 (taichi versus white crane)

After watching the YouTube movie many people were not impressed with the performance of the two famous masters, who had a secret gentleman's agreement not to use deadly moves to get a quick victory. They both knew that if any lethal move was used to beat the other guy there would be a lot of fights on the street among their students.

The Ji form of tai chi power can be cross-trained and enhanced by using tennis strokes. It is most obvious in my modified backhand:

The Ji form of tai chi power let you hit the ball in front of you easily.

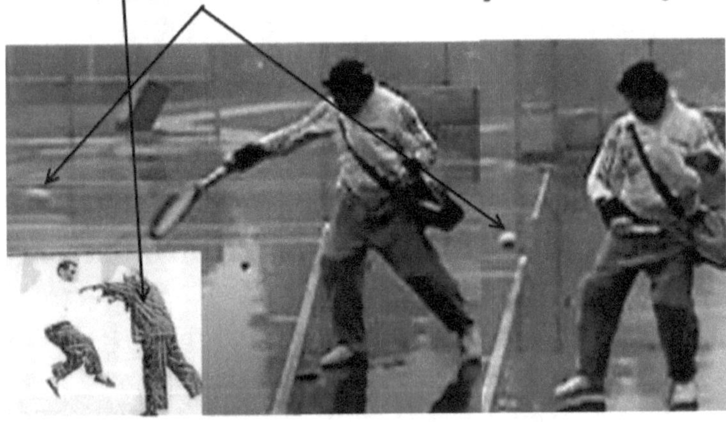

It can be used in the forehand too but it needs a higher skill level. You have to have a strong wrist because you have to flex the wrist backward to make an angle with the racket so that it can hit the ball in front of you. It is most useful when the ball hits you directly. This occurs most often in the return of serves when the opponent wants to jam you with a fast serve that hits at you directly instead of aiming at the corners.

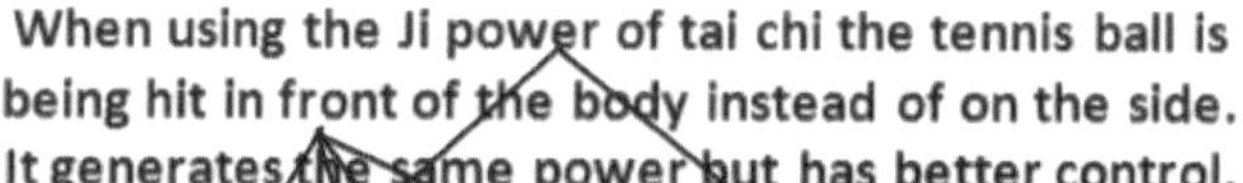

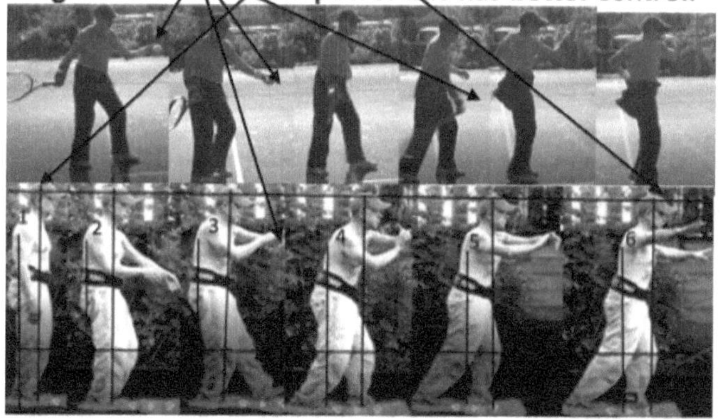

There is a YouTube movie on this:

https://youtu.be/U502VtqaCi8

Using tennis to enhance tai chi power and walking chanting meditation lesson by Dr. George Ho

I have made two YouTube movies showing my power of tai chi in a tennis serve.

https://www.youtube.com/watch?v=2UYWjLbd0V8&t=11s

Tai chi power and weight training as a form of IMBT (Integrative Mind Body Training)

https://www.youtube.com/watch?v=9_O6edSSRNg

An innovative program to train Dong jin 懂勁 in tai chi by Dr. George Ho

The above movies outline my new concept of teaching and training tai chi as a form of IMBT (Integrative Mind Body Training), which includes Dantian singing as a way to train Dantian breathing used in tai chi and qi gong.

Dantian breathing is best taught by Dantian singing because breathing is hard to observe and monitor but singing is not only easily audible, it can also be taught over the internet and one can also teach oneself with books and movies. The progress can be monitored easily.

In Vancouver I can teach an experimental class of tai chi tennis serve to test and monitor tai chi power.

To fully understand my article, "The Ji 擠 form of tai chi power compared with Bruce Lee's One-in-punch

Subtitle: The Ji 擠 form of tai chi power explained and trained scientifically", introduced in my YouTube movie with the same title, which can be used to search the aforementioned movie on YouTube, readers have to view the following links in the illustrations of the movie:

https://www.youtube.com/watch?v=2UYWjLbd0V8&t=11s

Tai chi power and weight training as a form of IMBT (Integrative Mind Body Training)

https://www.youtube.com/watch?v=eTOEjBWFr-8 鄭曼青 - 推手 **and the   push hand is at 2.37.**
https://www.youtube.com/watch?v=YdvrmvHA0ow&list=PL9RRMUY60ixTdZpWGySNpmYtCPSmegRpk&index=15

Singing the Silent Night as background music for doing the 4 forms of tai chi power by Dr. George Ho

• The Power of Internal Martial Arts and Chi: Combat and Energy Secrets of Ba Gua, Tai Chi and Hsing-I by

• Bruce Frantzis

 The link show of the cover of this book is http://www.barnesandnoble.com/w/the-power-of-internal-martial-arts-and-chi-bruce-frantzis/1111615333?ean=9781583941904

https://www.youtube.com/watch?v=ZRSAFG3QuVk

The tai chi 3/擠勁 (3/Ji jin) Ji power (energy) explained in the mystical dimension of Yi Jing 易經

https://www.youtube.com/watch?v=LPbKYpoIMEU

The Tai Chi CranioSacral Postural Reflex for better posture and tai chi (Copyrights reserved)

https://www.youtube.com/watch?v=3tTISzxQ86A

Tchoung Ta Tchen Push hands.m4v , published by Hamish Gordon in the YouTube channel on Dec 10, 2011.

Mr. Zhong Dazhen (鍾大振)wrote a tai chi book, 《太極拳體用注解》, which was written in both Chinese and English.

http://www.kamtotaichi.com/Chinese/aboutsifu/ctccac.html
http://www.jingwuhui.com/eshop/goods.php?id=4167

The demonstration of the explosive Ji power as shown in the above picture

http://taijiwenwutang.blogspot.ca/2006/02/blog-post_09.html

Wang 汪 Yongquan 永泉 (1903-1987)

https://www.youtube.com/watch?v=omDHWQLRSIc

☯ 牛春明大師 楊式太極拳 (完整版)

https://www.youtube.com/watch?v=3tTISzxQ86A

Tchoung Ta Tchen Push hands.m4v , published by Hamish Gordon in the YouTube channel on Dec 10, 2011.

http://taijiwenwutang.blogspot.ca/2006/02/blog-post_09.html

https://www.youtube.com/watch?v=O0Z3Zhj8ICY

太极拳之"千斤坠"，不知道外国人看到这个会相信么？

https://www.amazon.ca/Tao-Tai-Kung-Robert-Sohn/dp/0892812176

Tao and T'ai Chi Kung Paperback – Feb 1 1990

by Robert C. Sohn (Author)

https://www.youtube.com/watch?v=2FsZyPjsjTA

wu vs chan 1954 (taichi versus white crane)

At 8.10-8.11

https://www.youtube.com/watch?v=2FsZyPjsjTA

wu vs chan 1954 (taichi versus white crane)

At 8.10-8.11

https://www.youtube.com/watch?v=2UYWjLbd0V8&t=11s

Tai chi power and weight training as a form of IMBT (Integrative Mind Body Training)

https://www.youtube.com/watch?v=NCfWlYLKJLQ

Bruce lee's one inch punch

https://www.youtube.com/watch?v=pC6vRJsBZEg

Bruce Lee One and Six Inch Punches Slowed Down

https://youtu.be/U502VtqaCi8

Using tennis to enhance tai chi power and walking chanting meditation lesson by Dr. George Ho

Conclusion: This booklet has demystified the invincibility of tai chi as a form of martial art. The reason why some tai chi masters like the founder of Yang style tai chi or the founder of Sun style tai chi could easily defeat their opponents is not the special moves of tai chi it was their acquisition of the premonition power from the static Jing gong practice, like standing meditation, called 站椿 Zhàn zhuāng, reinforced and strengthened by the Dong gong practice of tai chi. This also explains why out of millions of contemporary martial art fanatics, like Bruce Lee there is not a single one who can defeat opponents like Yang Luchan and Sun Lutang.

Master Sun Lutang
Static
meditation
like 站椿
Zhàn zhuāng was
probably how he
acquired the
premonition
power that
made him
invicible like
Yang Luchan

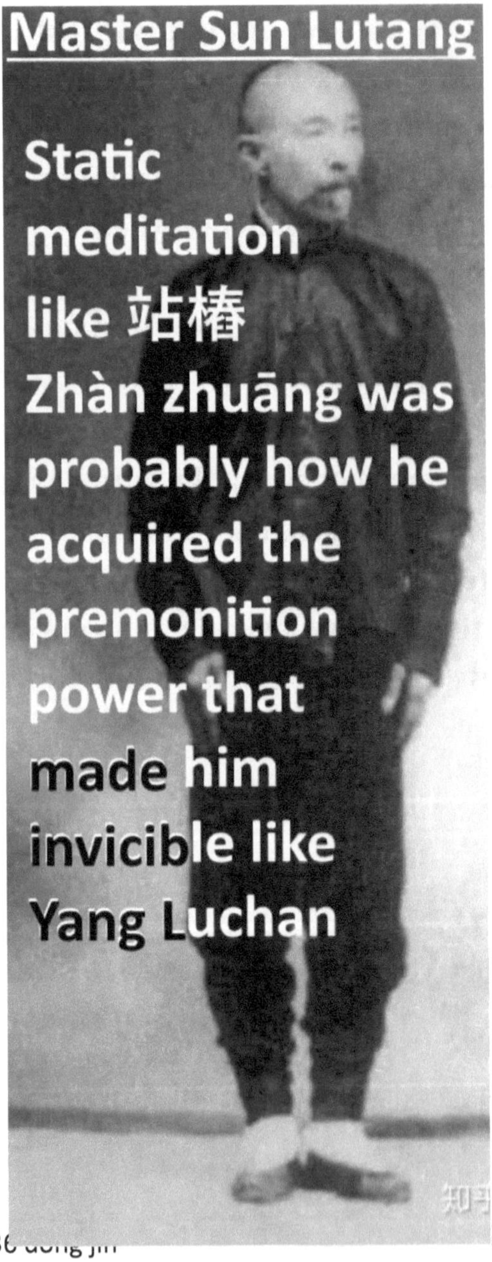

Static

meditation like 站樁 Zhàn zhuāng is hardly being emphasized in modern and highly commercialized martial art and tai chi instructions. In our highly commercialized age, nobody will pay instruction fees for years just to learn standing meditation.

In order to win the confidence of prospective students instructors like Yang 楊 shǎo hóu 少侯, the son of Yang Luchan had to use the most powerful form of tai chi power, the Ji power to push a partner flying up in the air, a show of power that could only be seen in a staged demonstration. From this finding, I have further developed the combination practice of Dong gong like tennis serves and walking with the principles of tai chi, combined with Jing gong like, "Sleeping qigong", handed downed to us from Master Chén tuán 陳搏 (AD 871-989) of the 宋 Dynasty in China.

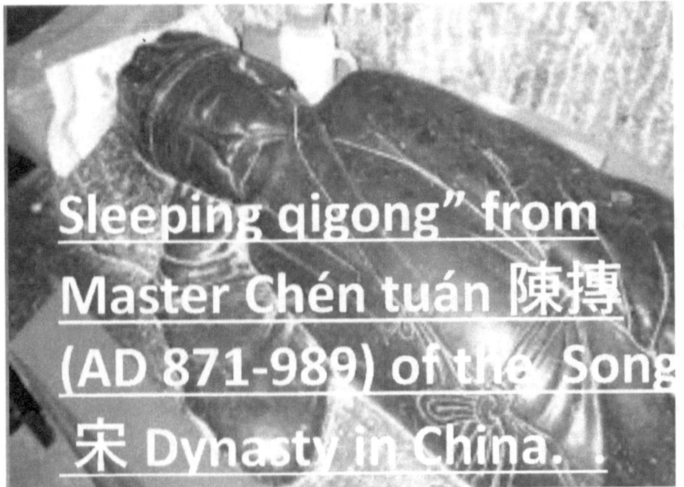

My books in Amazon.ca can be searched at:

https://www.amazon.ca/s/ref=nb_sb_noss_1?url=search-alias%3Daps&field-keywords=george+ho

1.The Dantian's Anatomy and Functions Explained Medically by Dr. George Ho

The link to the ebook in **Amazon.ca** followed by the abstract of this ebook:

https://www.amazon.ca/dp/B07GSJT8G7/ref=sr_1_2?ie=UTF8&qid=1535075597&sr=8-2&keywords=george+ho

Related supplemental YouTube video:

https://www.youtube.com/watch?v=LXuOjJfQ_Vc&index=8&list=PL9RRMUY60ixRHjIpvRSXudWjBVJF2rbkF

2.Can Tai Chi be self-learned? (Tai Chi and meditation by Dr. George Ho Book 1)

The link to this book:

https://www.amazon.ca/Benefits-tai-chi-spine-CranioSacral-ebook/dp/B07D8GVFCY/ref=sr_1_6?ie=UTF8 &qid=1530421365&sr=8-6&keywords=george+ho

Related supplemental YouTube video:

https://www.youtube.com/watch?v=xQK0EnXWz4M&list=PL9RRMUY60ixRHjIpvRSXudWjBVJF2rbkF&index=2

Self-taught tai chi? Answer in Kindle by Dr. George Ho

3.The Benefits of tai chi for the spine: The postural enhancement effect of tai chi, called the CranioSacral Postural reflex of Tai Chi (Tai chi and meditation Book 2)

The link to this book:

https://www.amazon.ca/Benefits-tai-chi-spine-CranioSacral-ebook/dp/B07D8GVFCY/ref=sr_1_3?s=digital-text&ie=UTF8&qid=1537985769&sr=1-3&keywords=george+ho

Related supplemental YouTube video:

4.The path to Enlightenment from the practice of Tai Chi + 站椿 Zhàn zhuāng (pile stance): Shen Ming is the Enlightenment Stage of Tai Chi, Superior to the ... Dong Jin" (tai chi and meditation Book 3)

The link to this book:

The path to Enlightenment from the practice of Tai Chi + 站椿 Zhàn zhuāng (pile stance): The Shen Ming of Tai Ch is the complementary component of your meditation for Enlightenment

https://www.amazon.ca/Enlightenment-practice-站椿 Zhàn-zhuāng-stance/dp/1983262641/ref=sr_1_10?ie=UTF8&qid=1537985438&sr=8-10&keywords=george+ho

Related supplemental YouTube video:
https://www.youtube.com/watch?v=CRpFxoWD41w&index=4&list=PL9RRMUY60ixRHjIpvRSXudWjBVJF2rbkF

The path to Enlightenment from the practice of Tai Chi + 站椿 Zhàn zhuāng (pile stance)

5.Treadmill Ram Tai Chi (TRTC): Chan (Zen in Japanese) walking with the breathing practice for health and longevity by Huai-jin Nan and Dr. George Ho (tai chi and meditation Book 4)

The link to this book:

https://www.amazon.ca/Treadmill-Ram-Tai-Chi-TRTC-ebook/dp/B07GJXGMWZ/ref=sr_1_5?s=digital-text&ie=UTF8&qid=1537985769&sr=1-5&keywords=george+ho

The related supplemental YouTube video:
https://www.youtube.com/watch?v=qEGjemhyvNc&index=1&list=PL9RRMUY60ixRHjIpvRSXudWjBVJF2rbkF

Chan (Zen in Japanese) walking can enhance the function of the kidneys

https://www.youtube.com/watch?v=UwJW0rjU kFY&list=PL9RRMUY60ixRHjIpvRSXudWjB VJF2rbkF&index=3

6.The Ji 擠 form of tai chi power compared with Bruce Lee's One-in-punch: The Ji 擠 form of tai chi power explained and trained scientifically (tai chi and meditation Book 5)

The link to this book:

https://www.amazon.ca/Benefits-tai-chi-spine-CranioSacral-ebook/dp/B07D8GVFCY/ref=sr_1_3?s=digital-text&ie=UTF8&qid=1537985769&sr=1-3&keywords=george+ho

Related supplemental YouTube video:

https://www.youtube.com/watch?v=51-pTS2-JxM&list=PL9RRMUY60ixRHjIpvRSXudWjBVJF2rbkF&index=6

The Ji 擠 form of tai chi power compared with Bruce Lee's One-in-punch

143 dong jin

7.Dolphin Instant Tai Chi

This link to this book:

https://www.amazon.ca/Dolphin-Instant-Tai-Chi-George-ebook/dp/B07G459TYR/ref=sr_1_8?s=digital-text&ie=UTF8&qid=1537985769&sr=1-8&keywords=george+ho

Related supplemental YouTube video:

https://www.youtube.com/watch?v=mK8pnjf_hDQ&index=5&list=PL9RRMUY60ixRHjIpvRSXudWjBVJF2rbkF

**THE EASIEST TAI CHI TO LEARN,
"Dolphin Instant Tai Chi"**

8.Meditation Bliss and Physical Health with Chan Walking and Swimming for All, including the Disabled

**Amazon.ca's Kindle book link:
https://www.amazon.ca/dp/B07H1NWB51/ref=s
r_1_2?ie=UTF8&qid=1535947626&sr=8-
2&keywords=george+ho**

Related supplemental YouTube video:

**https://www.youtube.com/watch?v=4HlvOa2X
Lkc&list=PL9RRMUY60ixRHjIpvRSXudWjB
VJF2rbkF&index=9**

**Meditation Bliss and Physical Health with
Chan Walking and Swimming for All, including
the Disabled**

**9.Prof. Lin Jùnqīng's 8 Steps of the Pharyngeal
Voice Training** 林俊卿博士（咽音練聲法的八
個步驟）

**The link to this book:
https://www.amazon.ca/Prof-Jùnqīngs-Steps-
Pharyngeal-Training-
ebook/dp/B07HDYSW5H/ref=sr_1_1?s=digital-
text&ie=UTF8&qid=1537985769&sr=1-
1&keywords=george+ho**

His writing in Chinese is available free on the internet by searching with " 林俊卿博士（咽音練聲法的八個步驟）"□

Related supplemental YouTube video:

Kindle: Prof. Lin Jùnqīng's 8 Steps of the Pharyngeal Voice Training 林俊卿博士（咽音練聲法的八個步驟）

Prof. Line's original writing has been translated into English by Dr. George Ho of Vancouver and it has been published in Kindle.

10.The rehab exercise for "TFCC self-treatment" ebook at Amazon.ca by Dr. George Ho

The link to this book: https://www.amazon.ca/TFCC-Self-treatment-George-Kam-Ho-ebook/dp/B07D278WVV/ref=sr_1_11?s=digital-text&ie=UTF8&qid=1537985769&sr=1-11&keywords=george+ho

Related supplemental YouTube video:

**https://www.youtube.com/watch?v=b_Ox_HaZ
Sc0**

**The rehab exercise for "TFCC self-treatment"
ebook at Amazon.ca by Dr. George Ho**

**11. The Correct Interpretations of Two
Important Tai Chi Concepts: "鬆開 Song kai"
by Yang Chengfu 楊澄甫 and Peng jin 弸 勁,
the Peng form of concentrated Tai Chi power**

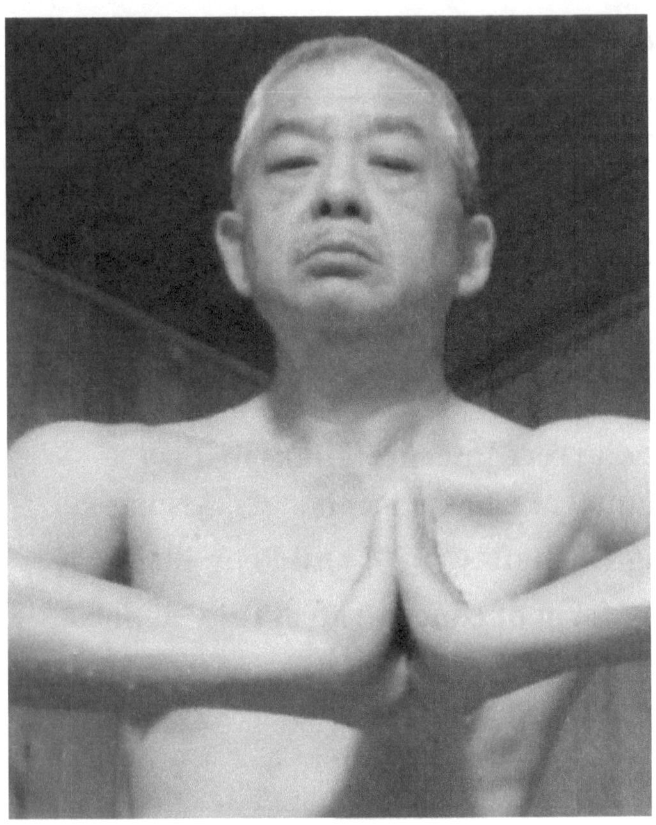

148 dong jin

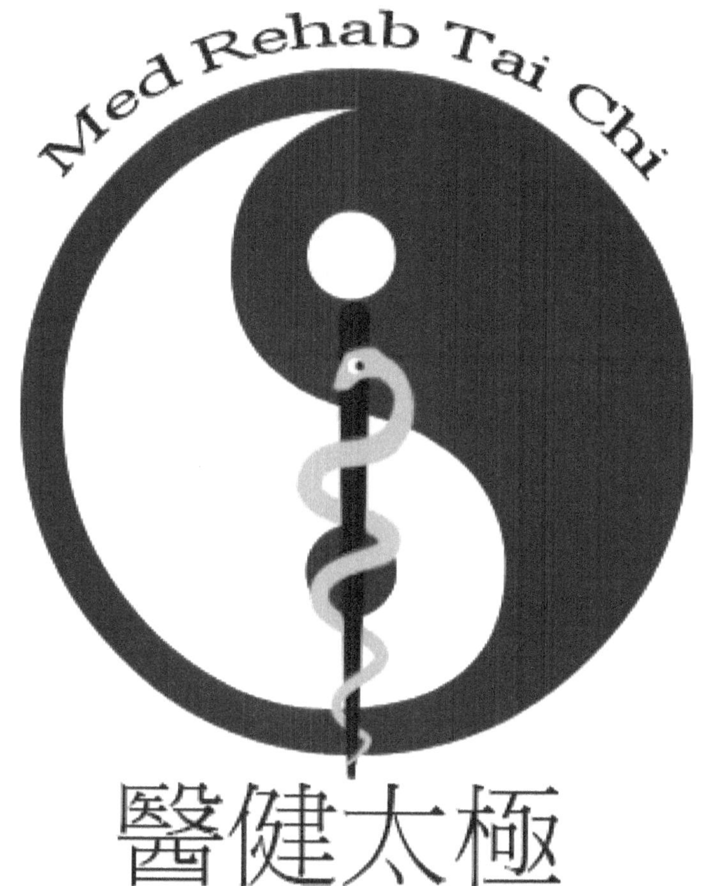

醫健太極

以<u>醫學</u>知識解釋太極／樁功／氣功／坐禪的療效以<u>科學</u>方法為訓練宗旨，將先賢文化發揚光大

**The Therapeutic Value of
TaiChi/Yoga/Qigong/Zen Explained <u>Medically</u>
and Trained <u>Scientifically</u>**

**My book, Med Rehab Tai Chi (MRTC)
ISBN <u>978-0-9866170-0-3</u> was published in the
：Summer of 2010**

**Place of publication: 5291 Hummingbird Dr,
Richmond, B.C. Canada, V7E 5T7
*(Georgekwho@yahoo.com)***

**Self-publishing author: Dr. George Ho,
B.Soc.Sc., M.A., D.C.**

---

[i] 鄭, 曼青. *鄭子太極拳十三篇*. 台北: 大展出版社, 1992. Print. P.53

Zheng, Manqing. *T'ai chi ch'uan a simplified method of calisthenics for health & self-defense.* Richmond, Calif: North Atlantic Books, 1981. Print.

Dr. George Ho's publications in English:

I have the following articles in scanned pdf format available online.

Articles in English:

To buy the article pay US$ 5 to the PayPal account, Georgekwho@gmail.com. After payment the article in scanned pdf format will be sent out by e-mail from Vancouver:

1/"The Anatomical Definition of the Dantian and a scientific definition of Qi that can explain why many famous Tai Chi masters are obese with excessive visceral fat" in scanned pdf format. https://www.youtube.com/watch?v=UbVyUo16nw4

2/The Tai Chi CranioSacral Postural Reflex for better posture and tai chi (Copyrights reserved)" https://www.youtube.com/watch?v=LPbKYpoIMEU

3/ "A Non-invasive Cure of Plantar Fasciitis" (All copyrights reserved) https://www.youtube.com/watch?v=2J_HQ9y2xOM

4/ "The TFCC ,Triangular Fibrocartilage Complex, home therapy with no drug or surgery "in scanned pdf format. https://www.youtube.com/watch?v=P-6aEOCGQQc

5/"A Non-drug, Non-surgery Tennis Elbow Cure" https://www.youtube.com/watch?v=9g7gjWw0JyY&index=5&list=PL9RRMUY60ixTvXmr6dKYQU9GGdhx-7G1n

6/ "The Innovative Self-management of Sacroiliac joint dysfunction; one-sided buttock back pain"
https://www.youtube.com/watch?v=NGL4G0kMSVg&index=6&list=PL9RRMUY60ixTvXmr6dKYQU9GGdhx-7G1n

7/"Beyond Relaxation" in tai chi
https://www.youtube.com/watch?v=OJVbymIYjQM&t=1s

8/Shen Ming 神明 is the Mental Enrichment Stage of Tai Chi by Dr. George Ho

https://www.youtube.com/watch?v=2R268Ermjwg

9/ The Ji 擠 form of tai chi power explained and trained scientifically

https://www.youtube.com/watch?v=CJ1maumh8po
10/Tai chi and spine

https://www.youtube.com/watch?v=8biT_HM3

<u>**VO0**</u>

11/Treadmill Ram Tai Chi

<u>https://www.youtube.com/watch?v=5Wd4iJaQ3GA&list=PL9RRMUY60ixRiQaFv1jKTqhDQRNbxeADF&index=16</u>

12/Excel on your own in Tai Chi as a form of Integrative Mind Body Training

<u>https://www.youtube.com/edit?video_id=FSmfiGaQf9c</u>

13/Dolphin Instant Tai Chi

<u>https://www.youtube.com/edit?video_id=lI7djPYR0_8</u>

• 想自療以下健康問題者,請購買在下的文章, 線上購買文章(scanned pdf format) 途徑: 費用:美金 US$5 元,用 PayPal a/c:, 付款給 Georgekwho@gmail.com,收到付款+電郵地址後便從溫哥華電郵出文章。可通過電郵

Georgekwho@gmail.com 接觸筆者。

第一篇中文文章

治大肚腩: 1/"丹田、命門的生理解剖和練法介紹: 以氣的科學定義解釋為何太極名師多大肚腩(練丹田的壞副作 用)?及防治大肚腩方法 "https://www.youtube.com/watch?v=TusZYhsxABA&list=TLGQaXtuokbNs

第 2 篇文章

治足底筋膜炎: 購買每一篇文章(scanned pdf format) 途徑: 購買自療足底筋膜炎 https://www.youtube.com/watch?v=LJ8h1RP7Le8&list=TLGQaXtuokbNs

第 3 篇教減肥

治高血壓高血糖: /"非藥物高血壓高血糖綜合療法"已出版兩篇文章

-

https://www.youtube.com/watch?v=um0F3H8s

TFA

第 4 篇文章

治媽媽手,腱鞘炎: 文章名:治媽媽手,腱鞘炎,購文章途徑

https://www.youtube.com/watch?v=84VVEoZuVrg&list=TLGQaXtuokbNs

第 5 篇文章

治尾指側手腕痛: "非手術非藥物尾指 側手腕痛自療法

https://www.youtube.com/watch?v=smbv9wxxfc8

第 6 篇文章解釋

練太極拳治壞姿勢之原理: "氣貼背頂頭懸合乎現代醫學解釋之丹田強脊健體法"

https://www.youtube.com/watch?v=9GPPO2UugGI

第 7 篇文章治單側腰眼部位的腰痛: :"創新非手術非藥物骶髂關節綜合症結合診斷治療的療法

"https://www.youtube.com/watch?v=aIjQXJ3N
Zxo

https://www.youtube.com/watch?v=rD_5ADuR
48Y

第 8 篇文章

治網球肘: 網球肘綜合療法

"https://www.youtube.com/watch?v=Wy-
IpGR916o&list=TLGQaXtuokbNs&index=12
附氣貼背照片,速治高爾夫球肘(肘隧道症)其他
腱鞘炎如腕管綜合症, 踝管綜合症 (腳踭內側痛),拇
指側手腕痛(俗稱媽媽手)腱鞘炎 ,扳機指治法的
介紹

第 9 篇文章治

足前掌痛: 足前掌痛(Morton's neuroma)莫頓氏
神經瘤的非手術非藥物療法

https://www.youtube.com/watch?v=0eOjCH4e
UQw

第 9 篇文章

<u>https://www.youtube.com/watch?v=abLW9Aw VZRc</u>

(粵)行禪唱誦壽而康又名跑步機之山羊太極丹田法 **by Dr. George Ho**

My YouTube channel:

Thanks you all for this 2943 subscriber's mile stone of my YouTube channel with   430,761 views and 2627 likes reached on 18th Nov., 2016.

The top ten movies getting some of the 2627 likes are:

1/Non-invasive cure of the piriformis syndrome by PNF (Copyrights reserved)

---

135 likes

2/(2)The Sacroiliac Joint Dysfunction Cure with an Innovative and Safe Self Treatment

55like

3/The tai chi 1/ 弸勁(1/Peng jin)Peng power (energy) explained in the mystical dimension of Yi Jing 易經

67likes

4/Curing lumbar disc hernia and acute low back pain (All copyrights reserved)

35 likes

5/The Dantian training secret in the old Cantonese opera tradition by Dr. George Ho

30 likes

6/(1 knee care) Smart care of the knee in exercises like Tai Chi and Qi gong

27 likes

7/The tai chi 2/ 捋勁 (2/Lu jin) Lu power (energy) explained in the mystical dimension of Yi Jing 易經

21likes

8/Practicing the first 5 basic forms of tai chi power with the 6 Healing sounds

19 likes

9/A supplemental movie to my first article of my Dantian and Mingmen' series (All copyrights reserved)

19 likes

10/Rejuvenation (4) Interpreting Master Huai-jin Nan's Anapana breathing technique

19 likes

A sequel to "Non-invasive cure of the piriformis syndrome by PNF stretching"(Copyrights reserved)

18 likes

The most popular playlists are:

 1/Tai Chi, Dantian and Mingmen

2/Dr. George Ho - English videos

3/The 8 forms of power (also been translated as energy) of tai chi

感謝大家的捧場,在下的 **YouTube** 頻道超越了 **2900** 定閱者的里程碑,

在 **2016** 年 **11** 月 **18** 日的記錄為 **2943** 定閱者, **430,761** 人次觀看。最多人喜歡的首 **15** 部電影

1/如何根治椎間盤突出症 **lumbar disc hernia** 和 急性腰痛 **acute low back pain (All copyrights reserved)**

302 喜歡

2/呵、呬、呼、嘻、噓、吹、除病「六字口訣」 的正確練法和讀音(據禪宗大師南懷瑾老師經驗)

173 喜歡

3/根治胃酸倒流, 胃痛和胃消化不良的運動療法

154 喜歡

4/Non-invasive cure of the piriformis syndrome by PNF (Copyrights reserved)

135 喜歡

4/(1 治膝痛關節炎)退化性膝關節炎和有關運動和練功的膝關節護理 **All copyrights reserved**

129 喜歡

5/用諾貝爾得獎的定律根治 "梨狀肌綜合徵" ,上集 **(All copyrights reserved)**

103 喜歡

6/消炎,固定和復健根治足底筋膜炎 (腳跟,腳底痛)

83 喜歡

7/The tai chi 1/ 弸勁(1/Peng jin)Peng power (energy) explained in the mystical dimension of

Yi Jing 易經

67 喜歡

8/非手術、非藥物、非按摩速效根治骶髂關節綜合症 **All copyrights reserved**

60 喜歡

9/(廣東話)最簡易的自製酸奶法 **(yogurt) by Dr. George Ho**

55 喜歡

10/(2)The Sacroiliac Joint Dysfunction Cure with an Innovative and Safe Self Treatment

55 喜歡

11/有功力的太極的預備式=站樁=禪定, **"**靜之則合**"**的無極狀態**(All Copyrights Reserved))**

46 喜歡

12/控制血糖於最佳水平可以減肥，防糖尿病，治血壓高，心臟病

44 喜歡

13/根治"梨狀肌綜合徵"的續集,另一 PNF 療法 (All copyrights reserved 保留所有版權）。

44 喜歡

15/太極八法之弸、捋、擠、 按、肘配呵、呬、 呼、 嘻、噓、吹、除病「六字 口訣」之練習

37 喜歡

電影清單受歡迎的次序排列依次為:

1/丹田面面觀(科學和客觀地)

2/Tai Chi, Dantian and Mingmen

3/Dr. George Ho - English videos

4/關節炎及傷痛系列

5/The 8 forms of power (also been translated as energy) of tai chi

6/老而彌堅壽更康

7/Self treatments of health problems, aches and

---

pain

8/非藥物非手術防治心血管病和糖尿病系列

9/太極網球'是多用途的身心綜合練習

**10/Practical tai chi tennis and tai chi golf
modernize tai chi into a form of IMBT
(Integrative Mind Body Training)**

• 想自療以下健康問題者,請購買在下的文章, 線
上購買文章**(scanned pdf format)** 途徑: 費用:美
金 **US$5** 元,用 **PayPal a/c:**, 付款給
Georgekwho@gmail.com,收到付款+電郵地址
後便從溫哥華電郵出文章。可通過電郵
Georgekwho@gmail.com 接觸筆者。

•

第一篇文章

治大肚腩: **1/"**丹田、命門的生理解剖和練法介
紹: 以氣的科學定義解釋為何太極名師多大肚
腩(練丹田的壞副作用)?及防治大肚腩方法
"https://www.youtube.com/watch?v=TusZYhsx

ABA&list=TLGQaXtuokbNs

第 2 篇文章

治足底筋膜炎: 購買每一篇文章(scanned pdf format) 途徑: 購買自療足底筋膜炎 https://www.youtube.com/watch?v=LJ8h1RP7Le8&list=TLGQaXtuokbNs

第 3 篇教減肥

治高血壓高血糖: /"非藥物高血壓高血糖綜合療法"已出版兩篇文章

- https://www.youtube.com/watch?v=um0F3H8sTFA

第 4 篇文章

治媽媽手,腱鞘炎: 文章名:治媽媽手,腱鞘炎,購文章途徑 https://www.youtube.com/watch?v=84VVEoZuVrg&list=TLGQaXtuokbNs

第 5 篇文章

治尾指側手腕痛：''非手術非藥物尾指 側手腕痛自療法

https://www.youtube.com/watch?v=smbv9wxxfc8

第 6 篇文章解釋

練太極拳治壞姿勢之原理："氣貼背頂頭懸合乎現代醫學解釋之丹田強脊健體法"

https://www.youtube.com/watch?v=9GPPO2UugGI

第 7 篇文章治單側腰眼部位的腰痛：:''創新非手術非藥物骶髂關節綜合症結合診斷治療的療法''https://www.youtube.com/watch?v=aIjQXJ3NZxo

https://www.youtube.com/watch?v=rD_5ADuR48Y

第 8 篇文章

治網球肘：網球肘綜合療法
''https://www.youtube.com/watch?v=Wy-IpGR916o&list=TLGQaXtuokbNs&index=12

附氣貼背照片,速治高爾夫球肘(肘隧道症)其他腱鞘炎如腕管綜合症, 踝管綜合症 (腳踭內側痛),拇指側手腕痛(俗稱媽媽手)腱鞘炎 ,扳機指治法的介紹

第 9 篇文章治

足前掌痛: 足前掌痛(Morton's neuroma)莫頓氏神經瘤的非手術非藥物療法
https://www.youtube.com/watch?v=0eOjCH4e UQw

Other self-published books and articles:

 - MRTC (Med Rehab Tai Chi)

- Dolphin Instant Tai Chi

- Treadmill Ram Tai Chi

-Joint and Related Problems of the Extremities (Hand and leg)

- People's Medicine (1): The Inspirational Case of Bill Clinton's Cure of his Heart Disease

- People's Medicine (2): Plantar Fasciitis

- People's Medicine (3) The Innovative Diagnosis and Treatment Combined Drugless and Non-surgical Therapy of Sacroiliac Joint Dysfunction

- People's Medicine (4) The Rejuvenation Manual (The Heart Rejuvenation Section);

- People's Medicine (5): Wrist Pain of the Ulna (pinky) Side

- Treatment of Tennis Elbow, a Comprehensive Approach

Profile of Dr. George Kam Wing Ho,

B. Soc. Sc., M.A., D.C.

Contacts: Cell. 778-840-4153, Georgekwho@yahoo.com

Facebook: http://www.facebook.com/georgekwho

Youtube: Uploads are accessible by keying in "Dr George Ho of Vancouver". Many of my videos will appear.

Skype ID: Georgekwho in Vancouver Canada

Vancouver Research and Teaching Clinic: 5291 Hummingbird Drive, Richmond, B.C. V7E 5T7, Ph. 778-840-4153

Working Experiences

-Associate at the chiropractic clinic of Dr. Ng Shu Yan in Hong Kong<ngshuyanhcc@gmail.com>,

1984-1985

-Registered member of the College of Chiropractors of B C

(http://www.bcchiro.com/)1985-2011

- Health columnist at a Hong Kong magazine, the Financial Trend (the publisher has closed down in 2007.)   1989-2006

-Director of Rehab Tai Chi Program and Honorary Medical Advisor of Vitality Tai Chi Academy, Ref. Tai Chi Master, Mr. Frankie Choi, email: "frankie choi" <funkien@telus.net>   1998- Present

-Registered chiropractor of Hong Kong Government Chiropractic Council, registered#CC000091   2006 till present

(http://www.chiro-council.org.hk/english/index_reg.htm);

- Finished an ergonomic project for the Canadian Consulate of Hong Kong. Reference available on request.   Jan 2008

-Being appointed as an Honorary Medical Advisor of 養生學會, Ref. Louis Tong, Director（www.islt.com.hk）

- Being invited as a guest speaker at Prof. Ceng-hua Long's lecture on the vertebrogenic origins of organic diseases at Stanford University Oct., 25,2009

Reference: Prof. Ceng-hua Long, cenghua long

longcenghua@163.com   (inquiry only in simplified Chinese please)   July 2008 – Present

-Presentation of an academic paper with Prof. Lorenz of Kent State University, "<u>Dantian Singing in Cantonese: A Theory about the Health Impact of Sound</u>" at the Sixth International Conference on Health, Wellness and Society on 21st Oct., 2016 in Washington D.C.

Please compare the following two pictures. In the 2016 picture Dr. Ho appeared younger than the 2009 one. It might be due to his rejuvenation practices.

Health, Wellness & Society Knowledge Community
Sixth International Conference on Health, Wellness & Society
Catholic University of America, Washington D.C., USA
20-21 October 2016
The International Journal of Health, Wellness, and Society
Volume 6, 2016
Knowledge Community Membership
20-21 Oct., 2016
Catholic University of America, Washington D.C.
"Dantian Singing in Cantonese: A Theory about the Health Impact of Sound"
Prof. Ralph Lorenz, Ph.D.
Dr. George K.W. Ho, D.C., M.A.

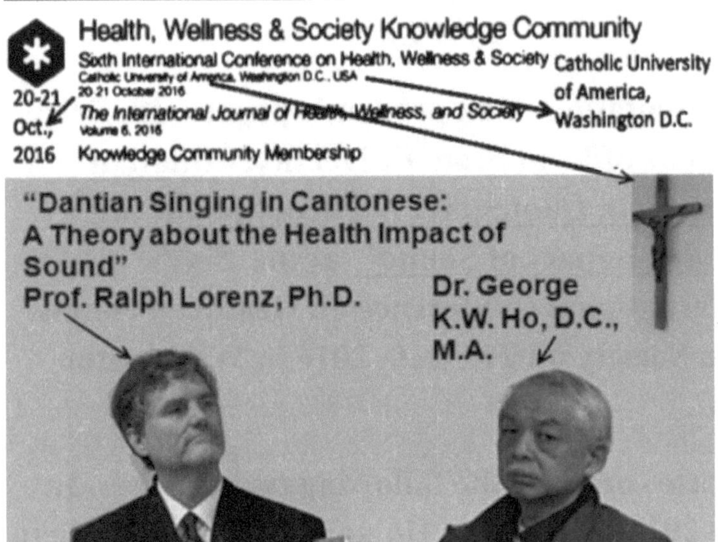

174 dong jin

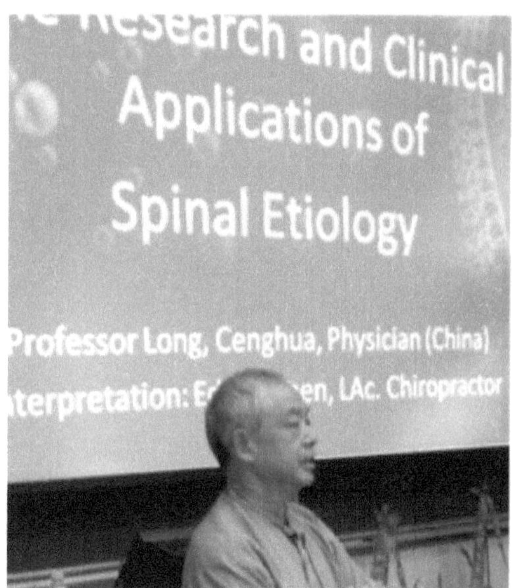

<-Dr. George Ho was invited as a guest speaker at Prof. Ceng-hua Long's lecture on the vertebrogenic origins of organic diseases at Stanford University Oct., 25,2009